Directory
of Health, Education,
and Research Journals

Lee Pratt

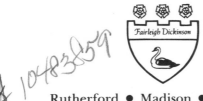

Rutherford • Madison • Teaneck
Fairleigh Dickinson University Press
London and Toronto: Associated University Presses

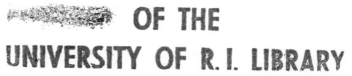

Associated University Presses
440 Forsgate Drive
Cranbury, NJ 08512

Associated University Presses
25 Sicilian Avenue
London WC1A 2QH, England

Associated University Presses
2133 Royal Windsor Drive
Unit 1
Mississauga, Ontario
Canada L5J 1K5

Library of Congress Cataloging in Publication Data

Pratt, Lee, 1934–
  Directory of health, education, and research
journals.

  Includes indexes.
  1. Medicine—Periodicals—Directories. 2. Health—
Periodicals—Directories. 3. Sciences—Periodicals—
Directories. 4. Research—Periodicals—Directories.
I. Title. [DNLM: 1. Health/Period Direct. 2. Education,
Medical/Period Direct. 3. Research/Period Direct—
periodical—directories. ZW 1 P915d]
R711.P74   1984   610'.5   83-49214
ISBN 0-8386-3213-0

Printed in the United States of America

Contents

Introduction   7

Alphabetical Listing of Journals   11

Indexes   123
  Professional Association   123
  Subject, Title, and Key Word   126

Introduction

RATIONALE
This research was initiated more than a year ago for my own professional growth. Since the emphasis today in education is directed toward research and publication, data collection began to extend my scope of research and publication options from the four journals within my file to a broader scope of possibilities.

The background of professionals in the health field includes a very heterogeneous mix of disciplines such as researchers, educators, practitioners, students and other scholars. This compilation of the more than 400 health-related journals and periodicals is intended to make tasks related to research and publication easier. The Professional Association Index, and the Subject, Title and Key Word Index were prepared to help you find journals best suited to your needs as an educator, researcher, and author in the health field.

DATA COLLECTION
Utilizing the library method, a list of more than 500 health-related journals and periodicals was compiled including the name of the journal, the address and the telephone number where available. This list of unlimited possibilities for health publication motivated a plan to make this information available to other health professionals interested in education, research and publication.

The data collection form was developed to obtain relevant information on each journal and sent with a letter to the publishers; both the form and letter are self-explanatory.

COMMENTS TO AUTHOR
Comments on this publication that may assist with a future updated form are welcome and may be sent to: Dr. Lee Pratt, Room 63-C 817 West Franklin Street, Richmond, Virginia 23284.

Directory
of Health, Education,
and Research Journals

Accident Analysis and Prevention
Year of Origin: 1968
Publisher: Pergamon Press Inc., Maxwell House, Fairview Park, Elmsford, New York 10523. Tel: 914 592 7700
Editor: Frank A. Haight, The Pennsylvania Transportation Institute, Research Building B, University Park, Pennsylvania 16802. Associate Editors: Hans C. Joksch, Herbert Moskowitz, G. M. Mackay.
Subscription Rate: $155 one-year, $295 two-year. Includes postage and insurance.
Circulation/Frequency: 1200/Bi-monthly
Pages Per Issue: 80–100
Author Payment: 25 complimentary reprints
Photo Policy: Black and White Glossies
Scope of Journal: This journal is designed to provide a wide coverage of all the general areas relating to accidental injury and damage, including the pre-injury and immediate post-injury phases. Published papers deal with medical, legal, educational, behavioral, theoretical or empirical aspects of transportation accidents as well as those occurring at work or in the home.

Action Newsletter
Year of Origin: 1960
Publisher: American College Health Association, 152 Rollins Avenue, Suite 208, Rockville, Maryland 20852. Tel: 301 468 6868
Editor: Kyle M. Johnson
Subscription Rate: Available Through Membership, Membership Fees Variable
Circulation/Frequency: Unavailable/10 yearly
Pages Per Issue: 8
Author Payment: None
Photo Policy: Photos Not Accepted

Writer's Guidelines: Contact Editor
Scope of Journal: This newsletter carries news and information of particular interest to health professionals at work in the college or university setting.

Activities, Adaptation and Aging
Year of Origin: 1980
Publisher: Haworth Publishing Company, 28 East 22nd Street
New York, New York 10010, Tel: 212 228 2800
Editor: Phyllis M. Foster, Activities Program Consultant, 6549 South Lincoln Street, Littleton, Connecticut 80121
Subscription Rate: $28 one-year Individual, $28 one-year Institution, $65 one-year Library
Circulation/Frequency: Unavailable/Quarterly
Pages per Issue: Variable
Author Payment: None
Photo Policy: Photos Not Accepted
Writer's Guidelines: Contact Editor
Scope of Journal: A professional periodical dealing with activities management with the increasingly aging American population. Emphasizes a multidisciplinary approach to concerns involving the aging that includes theory, research, case studies, specific programs and subsequent effects on the individual.

Addictive Behaviors
Year of Origin: 1975
Publisher: The Pergamon Press, Maxwell House, Fairview Park, Elmsford, New York 10523, Tel: 914 592 7700
Editor: Peter M. Miller, PhD
Subscription Rate: $95 one-year
Circulation/Frequency: 900/Quarterly
Pages per Issue: 200–240 average
Author Payment: None
Photo Policy: Photos Not Accepted
Scope of Journal: This journal is de-

signed to publish original research, theoretical papers, and critical reviews in the area of substance abuse. The journal focuses on alcohol and drug abuse, smoking and problems associated with eating.

Administration in Mental Health
Year of Origin: 1973
Publisher: Human Sciences Press, Box 2088, Rockville, Maryland 20852. Tel: 415 655 2801
Editor: Saul Feidman, D.P.A.
Subscription Rate: $23 one-year Individual, $48 one-year Institution
Circulation/Frequency: 2,000/Quarterly
Pages per Issue: about 175
Author Payment: None
Photo Policy: Photos Not Accepted
Scope of Journal: The aim of this journal is to advance the practice, study, and process of administration in the mental health setting. A major objective is to make mental health administration visible as a professional career and a field of knowledge and, by so doing, promote research and training programs. As a focal point for exchange and diffusion of knowledge, the journal seeks to foster communication and to enhance the vitality of mental health administration.

Administration of Social Work
Year of Origin: 1976
Publisher: Haworth Press, 28 East 22nd Street, New York, New York 10010. Tel: 212 228 2800
Editor: Simon Slavin, Ed.D., Hunter College, City University of NY, School of Social Work, 129 East 79 Street, New York, New York 10021. Tel: 212 570 5179, 914 949 8476
Subscription Rate: $36 one-year, $48 two-years, $65 three-years

Circulation/Frequency: 2,600/Quarterly
Pages per Issue: about 115
Author Payment: None
Photo Policy: Photos Not Accepted
Writer's Guidelines: Contact Editor
Scope of Journal: Publishes an array of articles, materials and announcements pertinent to administration of social work and human services.

Adolescence
Year of Origin: 1966
Publisher: Libra Publishing Co., Inc., 391 Willets Road, Roslyn Heights, New York 11577. Tel: 516 484 4950
Editor: William Kroll
Subscription Rate: $30 Institution, $25 Individual
Circulation/Frequency: 3,000/Quarterly
Pages per Issue: 256
Author Payment: Free Subscription
Photo Policy: Black and White Glossies or clear originals
Writer's Guidelines: American Psychological Association Style Manual
Scope of Journal: This journal is the result of our conviction that society's all too numerous failures in coping with the problems of adolescents stem from lack of coordination among the various professional disciplines: Psychiatry, psychology, physiology, sociology, education. Consequently, the main objective is the achievement of such coordination rather than the presentation of a specific point of view. Contains book reviews as well.

Advances in Alcohol and Substance Abuse
Year of Origin: 1978
Publisher: Haworth Publishing Company, 28 East 22nd Street, New York, New York 10010. Tel: 212 228 2800

Editor: Barry Stimmel, Dean for Academic Affairs, Mt. Sinai School of Medicine, Annenberg 5, 1 Gustave L. Levy Place, New York, New York 10029
Subscription Rate: $45 one-year Individual, $60 one-year Institution $90 one-year Library
Circulation/Frequency: 2,022/Quarterly
Pages per Issue: Variable
Author Payment: None
Photo Policy: Photos Not Accepted
Writer's Guidelines: Contact Editor
Scope of Journal: Each issue covers a single area in-depth with an emphasis on critical and synthesizing literature reviews of current knowledge in the field, and practical implications for treatment.

Advances in Behavior Research and Therapy

Year of Origin: 1978
Publisher: Pergamon Press, Maxwell House, Fairview Park, Elmsford, New York 10523. Tel: 914 592 7700
Editor: Professor S. Raehman, Department of Psychology, Institute of Psychiatry, De Criespigny Park, London, England
Subscription Rate: $85 one-year
Circulation/Frequency: 1,200/Quarterly
Pages per Issue: 780
Author Payment: None
Photo Policy: Photos Not Accepted
Scope of Journal: The aim of this journal is to encourage and facilitate the dissemination of new ideas, findings and formulations in the field of Behaviour Therapy. In particular, the editors hope to provide research and clinical workers with the opportunity to describe progress and convey their ideas in depth. The journal will publish papers that critically review a topic, present a systematic theoretical analysis or any integrated series of experiments.

African Journal of Medicine and Medical Science

Publisher: Blackwell Scientific Publications, Osney Mead, Oxford OX 2 OEL, England. Tel: 0865 40201
Editor: L. A. Salako, Dept. of Pathology, University College Hospital, University of Ibadan, Ibadan, Nigeria
Subscription Rate: $97.50 one-year USA & Canada
Circulation/Frequency: 490/Quarterly
Pages per Issue: about 75
Author Payment: None
Photo Policy: Black and White Glossies Accepted
Writer's Guidelines: Contact Editor
Scope of Journal: This journal serves as a forum for publications relating to conferences in medical sciences in Africa; to act as an exchange for information and opinions among medical scientists in Africa and elsewhere; to promote inter-regional cooperation amongst medical scientists in Africa and elsewhere; and to provide a medium for international dissemination of information about medical sciences in Africa and elsewhere.

Aging

Year of Origin: 1951
Publisher: Administration on Aging, 300 Independence Avenue SW, Washington, D.C. 20201. Tel: 202 245 1826
Editor: Jane B. Faris
Subscription Rate: $11 one year
Circulation/Frequency: 18,000/6 yearly
Pages per Issue: 48
Author Payment: None
Photo Policy: 5 × 7 Black and White Glossies
Scope of Journal: Geared primarily to service providers in the aging field but also accommodates researchers,

policy makers and the general public. Covers articles on new programs, legislation, surveys on segments of the elderly population, consumer-oriented issues, and how-to-do-it articles.

Alcohol Health and Research World
Year of Origin: 1973
Publisher: National Institute on Alcohol Abuse and Alcoholism, National Clearing House For Alcohol Information, Box 2345, Rockville, Maryland 20852. Tel: 301 468 2600
Editor: Margaret H. Hindman
Subscription Rate: $8.50 one-year, $10.65 one-year foreign
Circulation/Frequency: 7,000/Quarterly
Pages per Issue: 64 average
Author Payment: None
Photo Policy: Photos Not Accepted
Scope of Journal: Focuses on articles of interest to practitioners in alcoholism and related fields; includes literature reviews/state-of-the-art-articles, discussion of clinical experience, and research findings. Contains book reviews.

American Behavioral Scientist
Year of Origin: 1957
Publisher: Sage Publications, 275 South Beverly Drive, Beverly Hills, California 90212
Editor: Editorial Board. Contact: Sara Miller Mc Cune, Publisher and President
Subscription Rate: $22.50 one-year Individual, $44.10 two-year Individual, $65.70 three-year Individual, $49.50 one-year Institution, $98.10 two-year Institution, $146.70 three-year Institution
Circulation/Frequency: Unavailable/6 yearly
Pages per Issue: Variable
Author Payment: None

Photo Policy: Photos Not Accepted
Writer's Guidelines: Contact Editor
Scope of Journal: This journal is devoted to the enrichment of the social and behavioral sciences through interdisciplinary and policy-oriented interchange. Each issue focuses on those areas where several disciplines overlap . . . on areas where social science research has policy implications for social change . . . and on those problem areas emerging as fields for multidisciplinary behavioral study.

American Dental Association News
Year of Origin: 1970
Publisher: American Dental Association, 211 East Chicago Avenue, Chicago, Illinois 60611. Tel: 312 440 2782
Editor: Roger Scholle, DDS
Subscription Rate: $13 one-year USA, $24 one-year Foreign
Circulation/Frequency: 130,000/Monthly
Pages per Issue: 22
Author Payment: None
Photo Policy: Photos Not Accepted
Scope of Journal: The ADA News invited submission of articles, clinical reports, brief reports, reviews, perspectives, practice management, and conference summaries pertinent to dentistry and other health-related fields.

American Educational Research Journal
Year of Origin: 1964
Publisher: American Educational Research Association, 1230 17th Street NW, Washington, D.C. 20036. Tel: 202 223 9485
Editor: Gene V. Glass, Mary Lee Smith, Lorie Shepherd, University of Colorado, Boulder, Colorado 80309. Tel: 303 492 8609
Subscription Rate: $16 one-year Indi-

vidual, $21 one-year Institution, $12 one-year Members
Circulation/Frequency: 13,000/Quarterly
Author Payment: None
Photo Policy: Camera Ready Accepted
Scope of Journal: Contains original reports of empirical and theoretical studies in education. It is exclusively dedicated to publication of comprehensive reports of studies and of brief synopses of technical reports.

American Health: Fitness of Body and Mind
Year of Origin: 1982
Publisher: Owen Lipstein, 80 Fifth Avenue, Suite 302, New York, New York 10011. Tel: 212 242 2460
Editor: T. George Harris
Subscription Rate: $12 one-year
Circulation/Frequency: 400M/Bi-monthly
Pages per Issue: 96
Author Payment: None
Photo Policy: Photos Not Accepted
Scope of Journal: This journal is designed to deal directly with the current emerging lifestyle focused on individual health and well-being. Principal features cover recent developments in such areas as nutrition, fitness and exercise, prevention and psychology. Shorter items cover such topics as stress, new medical technologies, sports medicine and the economics of the health care system including the evaluation of doctors, drugs, insurance plans, etc.

American Heart Journal
Year of Origin: 1925
Publisher: C. V. Mosby Company, 11830 Westline Drive, St. Louis, Missouri 63141. Tel: 314 872 8370
Editor: Dean T. Mason, MD
Subscription Rate: $35 one-year Indi-

vidual USA, $56 one-year Institution USA, $28 one-year Student USA, $50 one-year Individual Foreign, $71 one-year Institution Foreign, $43 one-year Student Foreign
Circulation/Frequency: 12,000/Monthly
Pages per Issue: about 200
Author Payment: None
Photo Policy: Black and White Glossies
Scope of Journal: This journal will consider for publication suitable articles on topics pertaining to the broad discipline of cardiovascular diseases.

American Journal of Cardiology
Year of Origin: 1958
Publisher: Technical Publishing Company, 875 3rd Avenue, New York, New York 10022. Tel: 212 605 9400 or 212 605 9520
Editor: William C. Roberts, MD
Subscription Rate: $48 one-year
Circulation/Frequency: 25,000/12 yearly + special issues
Pages per Issue: 200–220
Author Payment: None
Photo Policy: Black and White Glossies, (Coloreds at Author's Expense)
Writer's Guidelines: Included in each journal
Scope of Journal: This journal is directed to publishing clinical research directed to the cardiologist and internists and includes brief reports and editorials.

The American Journal of Clinical Nutrition
Year of Origin: 1946
Publisher: American Society for Clinical Nutrition, Inc., 9650 Rockville Pike, Bethesda, Maryland 20014. Tel: 301 530 7110
Editor: G. M. Knight, Assistant Editor
Subscription Rate: $45 one-year Indi-

vidual, $50 one-year Individual Foreign, $60 one-year Institution, $65 one-year Institution Foreign, $17.50 one-year Student, $22.50 one-year Student Foreign
Circulation/Frequency: Unavailable/Monthly
Pages per Issue: 150–200
Author Payment: None
Photo Policy: 5 × 7 to 8 × 10 black and white
Scope of Journal: The primary purpose of this journal is to publish original research findings in the field of clinical nutrition. Perspectives in Nutrition, Editorials, Case Reports, special articles, and letters to the editor are also considered to be essential components.

American Journal of Clinical Pathology
Year of Origin: 1931
Publisher: J. B. Lippincott Company, East Washington Square, Philadelphia, Pennsylvania 19105. Tel: 215 574 4200
Editor: Myrton F. Beeler, M.D., Box 22, Louisiana State University Medical Center, 1542 Tulane Avenue, New Orleans, Louisiana 70112. Tel: 504 566 1487
Subscription Rate: $44 one-year Individual, $48 one-year Institution
Circulation/Frequency: 5,000/monthly
Pages per Issue: 50–70
Author Payment: None
Photo Policy: Black and White Glossies
Scope of Journal: This journal is devoted to prompt publication of original studies and observations in clinical and anatomic pathology. Original papers relating to laboratory use, management, and information science will be given consideration. A manuscript based primarily on data published previously is not acceptable.

American Journal of Community Psychology
Year of Origin: 1973
Publisher: Plenum Publishing Company, 233 Spring Street, New York, New York 10013. Tel: 212 620 8466
Editor: John C. Glidewell
Subscription Rate: $102 one-year USA, $115 one-year Foreign
Circulation/Frequency: unavailable/Bimonthly
Pages per Issue: 120
Author Payment: None
Photo Policy: large black and white glossies
Scope of Journal: This journal publishes an array of articles, materials, etc. pertinent to students and professionals in community mental health; contains book reviews.

American Journal of Digestive Diseases
Year of Origin: 1934
Publisher: Plenum Press, 233 Spring Street, New York, New York 10013. Tel: 212 620 8466
Editor: Frank Brooks, MD
Subscription Rate: $39.50 one-year Individual, $87.00 one-year Institution
Circulation/Frequency: 4,000/monthly
Pages per Issue: 70
Author Payment: None
Photo Policy: Black and White Glossies, (Colored at Author's Expense)
Writer's Guidelines: Guidelines Included In Journal
Scope of Journal: This journal will consider for publication suitable articles on topics pertaining to the title of this journal.

American Journal of Diseases of Children

Year of Origin: 1911
Publisher: American Medical Association, c/o Department of Pediatrics, University of Rochester Medical Center, Box 777, Rochester, New York, 14642. Tel. 716 275 2985
Editor: Gilbert B. Forbes, MD
Subscription Rate: $30 one-year, $56 two-year
Circulation/Frequency: 26,000/Monthly
Pages per Issue: 85–100
Author Payment: None
Photo Policy: Glossy Prints; Fee for Colored Slides
Scope of Journal: This journal publishes original articles, clinical memoranda, book reviews, special features of interest to students and professionals in the field of pediatrics.

American Journal of Epidemiology

Year of Origin: 1920 (formerly American Journal of Hygiene)
Publisher: The Johns Hopkins School of Hygiene and Public Health, 550 North Broadway, Suite 201, Baltimore, Maryland 21205. Tel: 301 955 3441
Editor: George W. Comstock
Subscription Rate: $60 one year
Circulation/Frequency: 4,000/Monthly
Pages per Issue: 150
Author Payment: None
Photo Policy: 8 × 10 Black and White Glossies
Scope of Journal: Publishes original contributions on epidemiologic research, demographic studies, case-control studies, etc., on diseases such as heart disease, cancer, stroke, hepatitis, influenza, congenital anomalies, as well as statistical or methodological articles. Reviews and commentaries on epidemiologic research are also published.

American Journal of Infection Control

Year of Origin: 1973
Publisher: The C.V. Mosby Company, 11830 Westline Industrial Drive, St. Louis, Missouri 83141. Tel: 314 872 8370
Editor: Mary Castle, RN, MPH, 1110 Glencoe Street, Denver, Colorado 80220
Subscription Rate: $34 one-year Institution USA, $37.50 International, $13 one-year Individual USA, $16.50 International, $10.40 one-year Student USA, $13.90 International
Circulation/Frequency: 6,540/Quarterly
Pages per Issue: 45
Author Payment: None
Photo Policy: Black and White Glossies
Scope of Journal: The official journal of Association for Practitioners in Infection 'Control. Articles submitted for publication should represent original communications related to the title and be submitted exclusively to this journal.

American Journal of Law and Medicine

Year of Origin: 1975
Publisher: American Society of Law and Medicine, Boston University School of Law, Boston, Massachusetts
Editor: Austin Stickells, J.D., LL.M., M.B.A., A. Edward Doudera, J.D., 765 Commonwealth Avenue, Boston, Massachusetts 02215. Tel: 617 262 4990
Subscription Rate: $40 one-year
Circulation/Frequency: 8,800/Quarterly
Pages per Issue: 150–200
Author Payment: None
Photo Policy: Photos Not Accepted
Writer's Guidelines: Contact Editor
Scope of Journal: The editors en-

courage the submission of manuscripts on a wide range of medicolegal topics. Acceptable subjects include: health law and policy; legal, ethical, social, and economic aspects of medical practice, education, and research; health-related insurance, etc. The journal is interdisciplinary and contributions from specialists in a variety of disciplines are welcomed.

American Journal of the Medical Sciences
Year of Origin: 1820
Publisher: Charles B. Slack, Inc., 6900 Grove Road, Thorofare, New Jersey 08086.
Tel: 609 848 1000
Editor: Saul J. Farber, MD
Subscription Rate: $35 one-year
Circulation/Frequency: 2,000/Bi-monthly
Pages per Issue: 68 maximum
Author Payment: None
Photo Policy: Two Sets of Unmounted Glossies
Scope of Journal: The purpose of this journal is to publish an array of articles on new material based on clinical or laboratory investigations in medicine and associated biologic disciplines.

American Journal of Medicine
Year of Origin: 1946
Publisher: Technical Publishing Company, 875 3rd Avenue, New York, New York 10022.
Tel: 212 605 9400
Editor: Arthur J. Antenucci
Subscription Rate: $46 one-year
Circulation/Frequency: Unavailable/Monthly
Pages per Issue: 150–200
Author Payment: None
Photo Policy: Black and White Glossies

Writer's Guidelines: Contact Editor
Scope of Journal: This journal publishes original scientific material including: case studies, seminars, hospital staff conferences, research, and symposia.

American Journal of Mental Deficiency
Year of Origin: 1876
Publisher: American Association on Mental Deficiency, 5101 Wisconsin Avenue NW, Washington, D. C. 20016.
Tel: 202 686 5400
Editor: Nancy M. Robinson, Child Development and Mental Retardation Center, WJ-10, University of Washington, Seattle, Washington 98195.
Subscription Rate: $45 one-year
Circulation/Frequency: 12,500/Bi-monthly July-May
Pages per Issue: 100 average
Author Payment: None
Photo Policy: Release Required
Scope of Journal: This journal is devoted to original contributions to knowledge of mental retardation and the characteristics of mentally retarded persons. Such contributions include reports of empirical research, tightly conceived theory papers, and systematic reviews of research literature on specific aspects of mental retardation. The preferred approach is objective, scientific, experimental, and theory-oriented.

The American Journal of Nursing
Year of Origin: 1900
Publisher: Thelma M. Schorr, RN
Editor: Mary Mallison, RN, 555 West 57th Street, New York, New York 10019.
Tel: 212 582 8820
Subscription Rate: $22 one-year
Circulation/Frequency: 365,000/Monthly

Pages per Issue: about 200
Author Payment: Upon Publication
$20/page less art and photos
Photo Policy: Black and White Glossies, Slides
Scope of Journal: It is the aim of this journal to present month-by-month the most useful facts related to health professions and especially to the field of nursing.

American Journal of Obstetrics and Gynecology

Year of Origin: 1920
Publisher: The C. V. Mosby Company, 11830 Westline Industrial Drive, St. Louis, Missouri 63141.
Tel: 314 872 8370
Editor: John I. Brewer, 710 North Fairbanks Court, Chicago, Illinois 60611.
Subscription Rate: 64.50 one-year Institution USA, $92.50 International, $43.50 one-year Individual USA, $71.50 International, $34.80 one-year Student USA, $62.80 International
Circulation/Frequency: 20,673/Semi-monthly
Pages per Issue: 130
Author Payment: None
Photo Policy: Black and White Glossies
Scope of Journal: This is the official publication for American Board of Obstetrics and Gynecology; The American Gynecological Society; The American Association of Obstetricians and Gynecologists and related state associations. Articles submitted must represent original communications related to the journal title and be submitted exclusively to this journal.

American Journal of Orthodontics

Year of Origin: 1915
Publisher: The C. V. Mosby Company, 11830 Westline Industrial Drive, St. Louis, Missouri 63141.
Tel: 314 872 8370
Editor: Dr. Wayne G. Watson, Box 1886, La Jolla, California 92038.
Tel: 714 459 1749
Subscription Rate: $52 one-year Institution USA, $64 International, $31 one-year Individual USA, $43 International, $24.80 one-year Student USA, $36.80 International
Circulation/Frequency: 14,373/Monthly
Pages per Issue: 125
Author Payment: None
Photo Policy: Black and White Glossies
Scope of Journal: The official journal of The American Association of Orthodontists, its Constituent Societies, and The American Board of Orthondontics. Articles submitted for publication should represent original communications submitted exclusively to this journal.

American Journal of Nursing

Year of Origin: 1900
Publisher: Thelma M. Schorr, President/Publisher, 555 West 57th Street, New York, New York 10019.
Tel: 212 582 8820
Editor: Mary Mallison
Subscription Rate: $120 one-year
Circulation/Frequency: 325,000/monthly
Pages per Issue: 200–250
Author Payment: None
Photo Policy: Black and White Glossies
Writer's Guidelines: Contact Editor
Scope of Journal: This is the official journal of the American Nurses' Association and includes an array of articles related to nursing. There are columns reporting news, medical highlights, and drug alerts.

American Journal of Orthopsychiatry
Year of Origin: 1930
Publisher: American Orthopsychiatric Association, 1775 Broadway, New York, New York 10019.
Tel: 212 586 5690
Editor: Edmund W. Gordon, Ed.D.
Subscription Rate: $20 one-year, $14 one-year student, $38 two-years
Circulation/Frequency: 13,500/Quarterly
Pages per Issue: 192
Author Payment: Pre-paid Subscription
Photo Policy: Photos Not Accepted
Scope of Journal: This journal is dedicated to informing public policy, professional practice, and knowledge production relating to mental health and human development, from a multidisciplinary and inter-professional perspective. Publishes articles and book reviews.

American Journal of Pathology
Year of Origin: 1901
Publisher: J. B. Lippincott Company, East Washington Square, Philadelphia, Pennsylvania 19105.
Tel: 215 574 4200
Editor: Donald B. Hackel, MD, F. Stephen Vogel, MD
Subscription Rate: $70 one-year USA Individual, $90 one-year USA Institution, $90 one-year Foreign Individual, $105 one-year Foreign Institution
Circulation/Frequency: 5,104/Monthly
Pages per Issue: Variable
Author Payment: None
Photo Policy: Photos Not Accepted
Writer's Guidelines: Contact Editor
Scope of Journal: Official publication of the American Association of Pathologists. Each issue contains firsthand reports on the major advances in the field of experimental pathology, and of new insights into basic disease processes.

American Journal of Physiology
Year of Origin: 1898
Publisher: American Physiological Society, 9650 Rockville Pike, Bethesda, Maryland 20014.
Tel: 301 530 7160
Editor: Stephan R. Geiger
Subscription Rate: $210 one-year USA, $240 one-year Foreign
Circulation/Frequency: Unavailable/Monthly
Pages per Issue: 600
Author Payment: None
Photo Policy: Black and White Glossies
Scope of Journal: This is the official journal of the American Physiological Society and publishes articles, reviews, experimental and theoretical studies, etc. of interest to all phsyiologists. Announcements are included of national and international meetings, career opportunities and reports of American Physiological Society affairs.

American Journal of Physiology: Cell Physiology
Year of Origin: 1887
Publisher: American Physiological Society, 9650 Rockville Pike, Bethesda, Maryland 20014. Tel: 301 530 7160
Editor: Stephen R. Geiger
Subscription Rate: $35 one-year USA, $45 one-year Foreign
Circulation/Frequency: Unavailable/Bimonthly
Pages per Issue: about 50
Author Payment: None
Photo Policy: Black and White Glossies
Scope of Journal: This journal is dedicated to the promotion of contemporary and innovative approaches to the study of cell and general physiology. It publishes original papers dealing with normal and abnormal cell function; manuscripts dealing with the structure and func-

tion of cell membranes, contractile systems, and cellular organelles, etc. Reports of research utilizing approaches including biochemistry, biophysics, molecular biology, morphology, and immunology are especially welcome.

American Journal of Physiology: Endocrinology and Metabolism

Year of Origin: 1887
Publisher: American Physiological Society, 9650 Rockville Pike, Bethesda, Maryland 20014. Tel: 301 530 7160
Editor: Stephen R. Geiger
Subscription Rate: $55 USA, $70 Foreign
Circulation/Frequency: Unavailable/Bimonthly
Pages per Issue: about 50
Author Payment: None
Photo Policy: Black and White Glossies
Scope of Journal: This journal publishes significant contributions to metabolic and endocrine physiology.

American Journal of Physiology: Gastrointestinal and Liver Physiology

Year of Origin: 1887
Publisher: American Physiological Society, 9650 Rockville Pike, Bethesda, Maryland 20014. Tel: 301 530 7160
Editor: Stephen R. Geiger
Subscription Rate: $50 USA, $65 Foreign
Circulation/Frequency: Unavailable/Monthly
Pages per Issue: about 185
Author Payment: None
Photo Policy: Black and White Glossies
Scope of Journal: Publishes original papers dealing with normal or abnormal function of the alimentary canal and its accessory organs including the salivary glands, pancreas, gallbladder,

and liver. Manuscripts dealing with digestion, secretion, absorption, metabolis, and motility relevant to these organs are encouraged. Reports of research utilizing techniques from other fields which contribute to the knowledge of physiology are welcome.

American Journal of Physiology: Heart and Circulatory Physiology

Year of Origin: 1887
Publisher: American Physiological Society, 9650 Rockville Pike, Bethesda, Maryland 20014. Tel: 301 530 7160
Editor: Stephen R. Geiger
Subscription Rate: $80 USA, $95 Foreign
Circulation/Frequency: Unavailable/Monthly
Pages per Issue: about 300
Author Payment: None
Photo Policy: Black and White Glossies
Scope of Journal: Publishes original investigations on the physiology of the heart, blood vessels, and lymphatics. The journal includes experimental and theoretical studies of cardiovascular function at all levels of organization. Preference is given to completed research which provides significant new insights. The journal publishes three types of articles: regular papers, rapid communications, and invited reviews.

American Journal of Physiology: Regulatory, Integrative and Comparative Physiology

Year of Origin: 1887
Publisher: American Physiological Society, 9650 Rockville Pike, Bethesda, Maryland 20014. Tel: 301 530 7160
Editor: Stephen R. Geiger
Subscription Rate: $40 USA, $50 Foreign
Circulation/Frequency:

Unavailable/Bimonthly
Pages per Issue: about 85
Author Payment: None
Photo Policy: Black and White Glossies
Scope of Journal: This journal publishes papers on broad and unifying themes of physiological science, focusing attention on relationships among components of physiological systems, on interactions among different levels within these systems, and on comparative physiology. Manuscripts which emphasize problems of communication and control are welcome.

American Journal of Physiology: Renal, Fluid and Electrolyte Physiology
Year of Origin: 1887
Publisher: American Physiological Society, 9650 Rockville Pike, Bethesda, Maryland 20014. Tel: 301 530 7160
Editor: Stephen R. Geiger
Subscription Rate: $60 USA, $75 Foreign
Circulation/Frequency: Unavailable/Monthly
Pages per Issue: about 200
Author Payment: None
Photo Policy: Black and White Glossies
Scope of Journal: Publishes original manuscripts that deal with renal or body-fluid and electrolyte physiology. Also, papers on broader aspects of excretion and secretion. Papers on the pathophysiology of disease of the kidney and of fluid and electroyle homeostasis are welcome. A special feature is invited reviews of a tutorial, research, and historic nature.

American Journal of Psychiatry
Year of Origin: 1844
Publisher: American Psychiatric Association, 1700 18th Street, NW, Washington, D. C. 20009. Tel: 202 797 4917
Editor: John C. Nemiah, M.D.
Subscription Rate: $35 one year, $48 one year Canada/Foreign
Circulation/Frequency: 35,000/Monthly
Pages per Issue: 150
Author Payment: None
Photo Policy: Photos Not Accepted
Scope of Journal: The official journal of the American Psychiatric Assoc. This journal publishes a number of peer-reviewed articles each month plus letters to the editor and book reviews. Articles should be directed toward the practicing psychiatrist and are both clinical and research oriented.

The American Journal of Psychotherapy
Year of Origin: 1947
Publisher: Association for the Advancement of Psychotherapy, Inc., 114 East 78th Street, New York, New York 10021
Editor: Stanley Lesse, MD
Subscription Rate: Contact Editor
Circulation/Frequency: 5,000/Quarterly
Pages per Issue: 150
Author Payment: Contact Editor
Photo Policy: Contact Editor
Scope of Journal: This journal is eclectic in which all aspects of psychotherapy and psychiatry are included. New research material is presented, together with critical evaluation of currently employed theories and techniques. Current literature is broadly covered: book reviews, review of literature, and an international section.

American Journal of Public Health
Year of Origin: 1911
Publisher: American Public Health
Association, 1015 Fifteenth Street
NW, Washington, D. C. 20005. Tel:
202 789 5666
Editor: Alfred Yankauer, MD, MPH
Subscription Rate: $50 one-year USA,
$60 one-year Foreign, $5 single copy
Circulation/Frequency:
35,000/Monthly
Pages per Issue: about 96
Author Payment: None
Photo Policy: Black and White Glossies
Scope of Journal: This is the official
Journal of the American Public
Health Association. Its primary purpose is to publish significant articles
covering the current aspects of public
health. Contributions are invited in
the form of original research and
evaluation studies, program evaluation of broad interest, and descriptive
analytic or methodological papers.

American Journal of Sociology
Year of Origin: 1895
Publisher: The University of Chicago
Press, 1130 East 59th Street, Chicago,
Illinois 60637. Tel: 312 962 8579
Editor: Edward O. Laumann
Subscription Rate: $50 Institutions,
$30 Individuals, $25 Students
Circulation/Frequency:
9,000/Bi-monthly
Pages per Issue: 260–270
Author Payment: None
Scope of Journal: This journal
"reflects a diversity of approaches
and concerns in all areas of sociology,
as well as perspectives from other social sciences, including psychology,
economics, statistics, anthropology,
history, political science and education." This publication contains approximately 50 pages of book reviews
and review essays as well.

**American Journal of Sports
Medicine**
Year of Origin: 1972
Publisher: Williams and Wilkins Company, 428 East Preston Street, Baltimore, Maryland 21202. Tel: 301 528
4133
Editor: Jack C. Hughston, M.D.,
American Orthopaedic Society for
Sports Medicine
Subscription Rate: $40 one-year USA,
$50 one-year Foreign
Circulation/Frequency: 9,000/monthly
Pages per Issue: 70–80
Author Payment: None
Photo Policy: Black and White Glossies
Writer's Guidelines: Contact Editor
Scope of Journal: This is the official
journal of the American Orthopaedic
Society for Sports Medicine and publishes all kinds of articles on injuries
related to sports.

American Psychologist
Year of Origin: 1946
Publisher: American Psychological Association, 1200 17th Street, NW,
Washington, D. C. 20036. Tel: 202
833 7686
Editor: Michael S. Pallak
Subscription Rate: Free With Membership, $50 Domestic Nonmember,
$54 Foreign Nonmember, $5 Single
Issue
Circulation/Frequency:
60,000/Monthly
Pages per Issue: 100–120
Author Payment: None
Photo Policy: Photos Not Accepted
Scope of Journal: This journal is the
official publication of the American
Psychological Association and, as
such, contains archival documents. It
also publishes articles on current issues in psychology as well as empirical, theoretical, and practical articles
on broad aspects of health.

American Rehabilitation
Publisher: Rehabilitation Services Administration, U. S. Department of Education, Room 3525, 330 C Street S.W., Washington, D. C. 20202. Tel: 212 264 4016
Editor: Ron Bourgea
Subscription Rate: $11 one-year
Circulation/Frequency: about 9,000/ Bimonthly
Pages per Issue: 32
Author Payment: None
Photo Policy: Black and White Glossies
Scope of Journal: This publication is interested in any kind of material related to rehabilitation of handicapped people that would be of interest to a professional audience i.e. educators, administrators, counselors, researchers. It accents direct language that communicates to a wide variety of readers.

American Review of Respiratory Disease
Year of Origin: 1917
Publisher: American Lung Association, 1740 Broadway, New York, New York 10019.
Tel: 212 245 8000
Editor: Gareth M. Green, M.D.
Subscription Rate: $90 one-year USA, Canada, Mexico, $100 one-year Foreign
Circulation/Frequency: 14,000/monthly
Pages per Issue: about 200
Author Payment: None
Photo Policy: Black and White Glossies
Writer's Guidelines: Included Within Each Journal
Scope of Journal: This is the official journal of the American Thoracic Society and embraces original articles concerning clinical, epidemiologic and laboratory studies of respiratory diseases. It also includes notes, correspondence with the editor, book reviews and official statements of the Society.

American Scientist
Year of Origin: 1913
Publisher: Sigma Xi, The Scientific Research Society, Inc., 345 Whitney Avenue, New Haven, Connecticut 06511.
Tel: 202 624 2566
Editor: Michelle Press
Subscription Rate: $20 one year, $35 two years, $45 three years, $3.75 single copy
Circulation/Frequency: 130,000/Bimonthly
Pages per Issue: 120
Author Payment: None
Photo Policy: Photos Not Accepted
Scope of Journal: This journal publishes articles that synthesize recent significant research findings, with enough background and interpretation to permit readers in other fields to understand them and appreciate their importance. The aim is to present articles by experts that describe the latest findings, with emphasis on their own research, in a way that will enable scientists outside the field to learn something about it.

The American Surgeon
Year of Origin: 1935
Publisher: J. B. Lippincott Company, East Washington Square, Philadelphia, Pennsylvania 19105.
Tel: 215 574 4216
Editor: Arlie R. Mansberger, M.D., Medical College of Georgia, Augusta, Georgia 30902.
Subscription Rate: $28 one-year USA, $34 one-year Foreign except Japan, $7 single copy
Circulation/Frequency: 3,511/Monthly
Pages per Issue: 40–60

Author Payment: None
Photo Policy: Black and White Glossies (Colored at Author's Expense)
Scope of Journal: This journal is designed for the publication of original articles dealing with clinical surgery. Emphasis and preference is given to material which surgeons can apply directly to the management of patients. It invites submission of papers which introduce new techniques or modifications of existing ones; deal with therapy which may include new anesthetic agents, diagnostic aids, care of infections; and which concern advances in knowledge of metabolism.

ASAIO Journal (The American Society for Artificial Internal Organs)
Year of Origin: 1978
Publisher: J. B. Lippincott Company, East Washington Square, Philadelphia, Pennsylvania 19105.
Tel: 215 574 4216
Editor: Dr. Pierre M. Galletti, 36 Taber Avenue, Providence, Rhode Island 02906.
Subscription Rate: $31 one-year USA, $35 one-year Foreign
Circulation/Frequency: 1,600/Quarterly
Pages per Issue: about 45
Author Payment: None
Photo Policy: Black and White Glossies
Scope of Journal: The ASAIO Journal will consider for publication manuscripts which describe the original research related to artificial organs of any type. Manuscripts can be submitted by members as well as nonmembers.

American Speech-Hearing Association Journal
Year of Origin: 1959
Publisher: American Speech-Language-Hearing Assoc., 10801 Rock-ville Pike, Rockville, Maryland 20852.
Tel: 301 897 5700
Subscription Rate: $50 one-year USA, $53 one-year Foreign
Circulation/Frequency: 43,000/Monthly
Pages per Issue: 80 average
Author payment: $65 page charge to author
Photo Policy: Camera Ready Accepted
Writer's Guidelines: American Psychological Association Style Manual
Scope of Journal: This journal is the house organ for the Association. It pertains to the professional and administrative activities of speech-language pathology, audiology, and the Association. Manuscripts may take the form of articles, special reports, news items, committee reports, book reviews, and letters. Articles should be of broad professional interest and may be philosophical, conceptual, historical, or synthesizing.

Anesthesiology
Year of Origin: 1940
Publisher: J. B. Lippincott Company, East Washington Square, Philadelphia, Pennsylvania 19105.
Tel: 215 574 4200
Editor: John D. Michenfelder, M.D., Department of Anesthesiology, Mayo Clinic, Rochester, Minnesota 55901.
Subscription Rate: $20 one-year USA, $50 one-year Foreign
Circulation/Frequency: 29,179/Monthly
Pages per Issue: about 60
Author Payment: None
Photo Policy: Black and White Glossies
Scope of Journal: Original articles with new information relevant to anesthesiology. Articles may deal with clinical material, applied research, or laboratory research. Also will consider

clinical reports, laboratory reports, reviews, medical intelligence, special articles and letters to the editor.

Annals of Surgery
Year of Origin: 1885
Publisher: J. B. Lippincott Company, East Washington Square, Philadelphia, Pennsylvania 19105.
Tel: 215 574 4216
Editor: David C. Sabiston, Jr., M.D., Department of Surgery, Duke University Medical Center, Durham, North Carolina 27710
Subscription Rate: $40 one-year Individual USA, $55 one-year Individual Canada/Foreign
Circulation/Frequency: 21,042/Monthly
Pages per Issue: 60–90
Author Payment: None
Photo Policy: Black and White Glossies up to 8 × 10
Scope of Journal: This journal considers publication of original articles in the field of surgery. It is the oldest continuously published journal in the English language solely devoted to the surgical sciences.

Annual Review of Biochemistry
Year of Origin: 1932
Publisher: Annual Reviews, Inc., 3129 El Camino Way, Palo Alto, California 94306.
Tel: 415 493 4400
Editor: E. E. Snell
Subscription Rate: $23 one-year USA, $26 one-year foreign
Circulation/Frequency: Unavailable/Yearly
Pages per Issue: 1,055
Author Payment: None
Photo Policy: Black and White Glossies
Writer's Guidelines: No unsolicited Articles
Scope of Journal: Hard cover periodical. Each issue is focused on a specific topic and contains 10 to 15 state-of-the-art reviews on current practice by leading specialists in the field. Unsolicited articles are not accepted. The "guest editor" of each issue invites papers on areas of current interest.

Annual Review of Genetics
Year of Origin: 1967
Publisher: Annual Reviews, Inc., 3129 El Camino Way, Palo Alto, California 94306.
Tel: 415 493 4400
Editor: H. L. Roman
Subscription Rate: $22 one-year USA, $25 one-year foreign
Circulation/Frequency: Unavailable/Yearly
Pages per Issue: about 500
Author Payment: None
Writer's Guidelines: No unsolicited Articles
Scope of Journal: Hard cover periodical. Each issue is focused on a specific topic and contains 10 to 15 state-of-the-art reviews on current practice by leading specialists in the field. Unsolicited articles are not accepted. The "guest editor" of each issue invites papers on areas of current interest.

Annual Review of Medicine
Year of Origin: 1950
Publisher: Annual Reviews, Inc., 4139 El Camino Way, Palo Alto, California 94306.
Tel: 415 493 4400
Editor: W. P. Creger
Subscription Rate: $22 one-year USA, $25 one-year foreign
Circulation/Frequency: Unavailable/Yearly
Pages per Issue: about 596
Author Payment: None

Photo Policy: Black and White Glossies

Writer's Guidelines: No unsolicited Articles

Scope of Journal: Hard cover periodical. Each issue is focused on a specific topic and contains 10 to 15 state-of-the-art reviews on current practice by leading specialists in the field. Unsolicited articles are not accepted. The "guest editor" of each issue invites papers on areas of current interest.

Annual Review of Microbiology
Year of Origin: 1947
Publisher: Annual Reviews, Inc., 4139 El Camino Way, Palo Alto, California 94306. Tel: 415 493 4400
Editor: M. P. Starr
Subscription Rate: $22 one-year USA, $25 one-year foreign
Circulation/Frequency: Unavailable/Yearly
Pages per Issue: about 560
Author Payment: None
Photo Policy: Black and White Glossies
Writer's Guidelines: No unsolicited Articles
Scope of Journal: Hard cover periodical. Each issue is focused on a specific topic and contains 10 to 15 state-of-the-art reviews on current practice by leading specialists in the field. Unsolicited articles are not accepted. The "guest editor" of each issue invites papers on areas on current interest.

Annual Review of Neuro-Science
Year of Origin: 1978
Publisher: Annual Reviews, Inc., 4139 El Camino Way, Palo Alto, California 94306. Tel: 415 493 4400
Editor: W. M. Cowan
Subscription Rate: $22 one-year USA, $25 one-year foreign

Circulation/Frequency: Unavailable/Yearly
Pages per Issue: about 392
Author Payment: None
Photo Policy: Black and White Glossies
Writer's Guidelines: No unsolicited Articles
Scope of Journal: Hard cover periodical. Each issue is focused on a specific topic and contains 10 to 15 state-of-the-art reviews on current practice by leading specialists in the field. Unsolicited articles are not accepted. The "guest editor" of each issue invites papers on areas of current interest.

Annual Review of Nutrition
Year of Origin: 1981
Publisher: Annual Reviews, Inc., 4139 El Camino Way, Palo Alto, California 94306. Tel: 415 493 4400
Editor: W. J. Darby
Subscription Rate: $22 one-year USA, $25 one-year foreign
Circulation/Frequency: Unavailable/Yearly
Pages per Issue: about 497
Author Payment: None
Photo Policy: Black and White Glossies
Writer's Guidelines: No unsolicited Articles
Scope of Journal: Hard cover periodical. Each issue is focused on a specific topic and contains 10 to 15 state-of-the-art reviews on current practice by leading specialists in the field. Unsolicited articles are not accepted. The "guest editor" of each issue invites papers on areas of current interest.

Annual Review of Pharmacology and Toxicology
Year of Origin: 1961
Publisher: Annual Reviews, Inc., 4139 El Camino Way, Palo Alto, California 94306. Tel: 415 493 4400
Editor: R. George, R. Okun
Subscription Rate: $22 one-year USA, $25 one-year foreign
Circulation/Frequency: Unavailable/Yearly
Pages per Issue: about 739
Author Payment: None
Photo Policy: Black and White Glossies
Writer's Guidelines: No unsolicited articles
Scope of Journal: Hard cover periodical. Each issue is focused on a specific topic and contains 10 to 15 state-of-the-art reviews on current practice by leading specialists in the field. Unsolicited articles are not accepted. The "guest editor" of each issue invites papers on areas of current interest.

Annual Review of Psychology
Year of Origin: 1950
Publisher: Annual Reviews, Inc., 4139 El Camino Way, Palo Alto, California 94306. Tel: 415 493 4400
Editor: L. W. Porter, M. R. Rosenzweig
Subscription Rate: $22 one-year USA, $25 one-year foreign
Circulation/Frequency: Unavailable/Yearly
Pages per Issue: about 744
Author Payment: None
Photo Policy: Black and White Glossies
Writer's Guidelines: No unsolicited articles
Scope of Journal: Hard cover periodical. Each issue is focused on a specific topic and contains 10 to 15 state-of-the-art reviews on current practice by leading specialists in the field. Unsolicited articles are not accepted. The "guest editor" of each issue invites papers on areas of current interest.

Annual Review of Public Health
Year of Origin: 1980
Publisher: Annual Reviews, Inc., 4139 El Camino Way, Palo Alto, California 94306. Tel: 415 493 4400
Editor: L. Breslow
Subscription Rate: $22 one-year USA, $25 one-year foreign
Circulation/Frequency: Unavailable/Yearly
Pages per Issue: about 496
Author Payment: None
Photo Policy: Black and White Glossies
Writer's Guidelines: No unsolicited articles
Scope of Journal: Hard cover periodical. Each issue is focused on a specific topic and contains 10 to 15 state-of-the-art reviews on current practice by leading specialists in the field. Unsolicited articles are not accepted. The "guest editor" of each issue invites papers on areas of current interest.

Applied and Environmental Microbiology
Year of Origin: 1953
Publisher: American Society for Microbiology, 1913 I Street NW, Washington D.C. 20006. Tel: 202 833 9680
Editor: James M. Tiedje
Subscription Rate: $120 one-year
Circulation/Frequency: 8,889/Monthly
Pages per Issue: 1,224
Author Payment: None
Photo Policy: Photos Not Accepted
Writer's Guidelines: Contact Editor
Scope of Journal: Both fundamental and applied aspects of environmental

microbiology are emphasized in this journal. It publishes descriptions of all aspects of applied research as well as both applied and basic ecological research on bacteria and other micro-organisms, including fungi, protozoa, and other simple eucaryotic organisms. Other topics that are considered are: microbiology in relationship to foods, agriculture, industry, and the public health and basic biological properties of organisms as related to microbial ecology.

Archives of Environmental Health
Year of Origin: 1945
Publisher: Heldref Publications, 400 Albemarle Street NW, Washington, D. C. 20016. Tel: 202 362 6445
Editor: Patricia M. Meyer
Subscription Rate: $40 one-year
Circulation/Frequency: 3,600/Bi-Monthly
Pages per Issue: 56
Author Payment: None
Photo Policy: Black and White Glossies 3 × 5
Scope of Journal: This journal publishes original research exploring the interface between medicine and the environment. The content of Archives of Environmental Health has value to scientists, physicians, and all individuals concerned with understanding the effects on health of toxic environmental substances. Contributors include well-known scientists working in the fields of academic medicine, public health, and biological and chemical research.

Archives of General Psychiatry
Year of Origin: 1959
Publisher: American Medical Association, 535 North Dearborn, Chicago, Illinois 60610. Tel: 312 751 6079
Editor: Daniel X. Freedman, MD, Box 2011, University of Chicago, De-partment of Psychiatry, Chicago, Illinois 60637. Tel: 312 947 1000
Subscription Rate: $30 one-year
Circulation/Frequency: 20M/Monthly
Pages per Issue: 70–80
Author Payment: None
Photo Policy: Black and White Glossies 5 × 7
Scope of Journal: Original articles dealing with advances in any area of psychiatry. Readership consists of practicing psychiatrists and mental health researchers. Letters to the Editor Section; No Book Review Section.

Archives of Sexual Behavior
Year of Origin: 1972
Publisher: Plenum Publishing Company, 233 Spring Street, New York, New York 10013. Tel: 212 620 8466
Editor: Dr. Richard Green
Subscription Rate: $110 USA, $124 Foreign
Circulation/Frequency: Unavailable/Bimonthly
Pages per Issue: 100
Author Payment: None
Photo Policy: Photos Not Accepted
Scope of Journal: This journal publishes an array of articles, materials and announcements pertinent to students and professionals in social sciences, health sciences and in particular sex therapy. Articles range from theoretical to case studies.

Arteriosclerosis: A Journal of Vascular Biology and Disease
Year of Origin: 1981
Publisher: American Heart Association, 7320 Greenville Avenue, Dallas, Texas 75231. Tel: 214 750 5300
Editor: Edwin L. Bieman, MD
Subscription Rate: $50 one-year USA, $65 one-year Foreign
Circulation/Frequency: 2,000/6 yearly
Pages per issue: Variable

Author Payment: None
Photo Policy: Black and White or
Color. Color Cost paid by author
Scope of Journal: This journal includes original research papers and
state-of-the art reviews from a variety
of disciplines bearing on the biology,
prevention, and impact of vascular
diseases relating to arteriosclerosis.

Association of Operating Room Nurses (AORN)

Year of Origin: 1963
Publisher: Association of Operating
Room Nurses, Inc., 10170 East Mis-
sissippi Avenue, Denver, Colorado
80231. Tel: 303 755 6300
Editor: Elinor S. Schrader
Subscription Rate: $35 one-year USA/
membership, $32 one-year Domestic/
Nonmember, $38 one-year
Foreign/Nonmember
Circulation/Frequency: 32,800/13
yearly
Pages per Issue: about 200
Author Payment: Honorarium: $5–
$25 per published page
Photo Policy: Black and White Glossies 5 × 7
Scope of Journal: This journal serves
as a means of communication to aid
in the successful accomplishment of
the aims and objectives of the Association of Operating Room Nurses.
The primary purpose of the AORN
is to provide assistance in the educational development of the operating
room nurse. It strives to provide
readers with practical and theoretical
information which will ultimately result in better patient care and im-
proved standards. It also publishes
current trends in the health care field
generally.

Australasian Nurses Journal

Year of Origin: 1964
Publisher: Messenger Publications,
254 Commercial Road, Box 197, Pt
Adelaide, Australia. Tel: (08) 475722
Editor: Edna Davis
Subscription Rate: $5 Australia, $10
Overseas
Circulation/Frequency: Unavailable/11
yearly
Pages per Issue: 32
Author Payment: Negotiable per
length
Photo Policy: Black and White Glos-
sies, 6 × 4
Writer's Guidelines: Contact Editor
Scope of Journal: Publishes nursing
studies, professional education, arti-
cles of human interest and worth-
while articles to nurses and other
health professionals.

Behavior Counseling and Community Interventions

Year of Origin: 1981
Publisher: Human Sciences Press, 72
5th Avenue, New York, New York
10011. Tel: 212 243 6000
Editor: John P. Galassi, Merna Dee
Galassi
Subscription Rate: $48 Institutional,
$24 Individual
Circulation/Frequency: 1,200/Bi-an-
nual
Pages per Issue: 64 average
Author Payment: None
Photo Policy: Black and White Glossies
Writer's Guidelines: No Specific
Guidelines; Use Format Within Journal
Scope of Journal: This journal provides an interdisciplinary forum to a
broadly conceived social learning orientation for counseling and commu-
nity-level interventions. Such an
orientation espouses the importance
of the scientific method, empirical

testing, and explicitly stated concepts and procedures. Articles on interventions, assessment, issues, theory, and reviews of the literature will be published for professionals interested in normal individuals coping with development concerns throughout life.

Behavioral Science
Year of Origin: 1956
Publisher: General Systems Science Foundation
Editor: James Grier Miller, University of California, Santa Barbara, California 93106. Tel: 805 961 2311
Subscription Rate: $25 one-year Individual, $40 one-year Institution, $35 one-year Foreign
Circulation/Frequency: 2,700/Quarterly
Pages per Issue: 400
Author Payment: None
Photo Policy: 8 × 10 Black and White Glossies
Scope of Journal: Interdisciplinary and conceptual articles on systems research, cross-level studies, new theories, experimental research, applications, modeling, and simulation.

Behavior Research and Therapy
Year of Origin: 1952
Publisher: The Pergamon Press, Maxwell House, Fairview Park, Elmsford, New York, 10523. Tel. 914 592 7700
Editor: Professor S. Rachman
Subscription Rate: $130 one-year
Circulation/Frequency: 3,500/Bimonthly
Pages per Issue: 600 average
Author Payment: None
Photo Policy: Photos Not Accepted
Scope of Journal: Contributions will stress equally the application of existing knowledge to psychiatric and social problems, experimental research into fundamental questions arising from these attempts to relate learning theory and maladaptive behaviour, and high level theoretical attempts to lay more secure foundations for experimental and observational studies along these lines.

Biofeedback and Self Regulation
Year of Origin: 1976
Publisher: Plenum Publishing Company, 233 Spring Street, New York, New York 10013. Tel: 212 620 8466
Editor: Albert F. Ax
Subscription Rate: $78 one-year USA, $88 one-year Foreign
Circulation/Frequency: Unavailable/Quarterly
Pages per Issue: 150
Author Payment: None
Photo Policy: large black and white glossies
Scope of Journal: Publishes an array of articles, materials and commentaries pertinent to students and professionals in health science . . . in particular biofeedback. Articles range from theoretical how-to-do-it; contains book reviews and abstracts.

Birth
Year of Origin: 1973–74
Publisher: Medical Consumer Communications, Inc., 110 El Camino Real, Berkeley, California 94705. Tel: 415 658 5099
Editor: Madeleine H. Shearer
Subscription Rate: $12 one-year Individuals, $18 one-year Institutions
Circulation/Frequency: 7,000/quarterly
Pages per Issue; 72
Author Payment: None
Photo Policy: Black and White Glossies
Writer's Guidelines: Included Within Journal
Scope of Journal: Professional journal of research and commentary on obstetric practices and directed to care of expectant parents.

Blood
Year of Origin: 1946
Publisher: Grune and Stratton, Inc., 111 Fifth Avenue, New York, New York 10003, Tel: 212 741 6800
Editor: Paul A. Marks, M. D.
Subscription Rate: $92 one-year USA, $96 one-year foreign
Circulation/Frequency: Unavailable/monthly
Pages per Issue: 250–300
Author Payment: None
Photo Policy: Black and White Glossies
Writer's Guidelines: Contact Editor
Scope of Journal: This is the official journal of the American Society of Hematology and includes research and commentary in the area of hematology; also reports business of the Society.

Breast Cancer Research and Treatment
Year of Origin: 1981
Publisher: Martinus Nijhoff, Box 566, 2501 CN The Hague, The Netherlands. Tel: 070 469 460
Editor: William L. McGuire, MD
Subscription Rate: $45.00 one-year Individual USA, $68.50 one-year Institutions USA, (Postage and Handling add $11 and Airmail add $9.50)
Circulation/Frequency: New/Quarterly
Pages per Issue: 80–100
Author Payment: None
Photo Policy: Photos Not Accepted
Scope of Journal: This journal creates a "market place" for breast cancer topics which cuts across all the usual lines of disciplines, providing a site for presenting pertinent investigations and for discussing critical questions relevant to the entire field. It aims to develop a new focus and perspective for all those concerned with breast cancer.

Briefs
Year of Origin: 1966
Publisher: Charles B. Slack, Inc., 6900 Grove Road, Thorofare, New Jersey 08086. Tel: 609 848 1000
Editor: Martin Kelly
Subscription Rate: $8 one-year
Circulation/Frequency: 2,100/10 issues a year
Pages per Issue: 16
Author Payment: None
Photo Policy: Photos Not Accepted
Writer's Guidelines: Follow Format Within Publication
Scope of Journal: This publication summarizes current literature in short article form on topics pertinent to maternity and neonatal health care.

British Journal of Addiction
Year of Origin: 1947
Publisher: Longman Group Ltd., Periodicals & Directories Division, 6th Floor, Westgate House, Harlow, Essex, CM20 1 NE England. Tel: 0279 442601
Editor: Griffith Edwards
Subscription Rate: $62 one-year USA Individual, free to members
Circulation/Frequency: 1,397/Quarterly
Pages per Issue: 450
Author Payment: None
Photo Policy: Photos Not Accepted
Writer's Guidelines: Contact Editor
Scope of Journal: This journal publishes original material, review articles and brief communications dealing with all aspects of alcoholism and drug dependence, and may also sometimes take papers on other compulsive behaviors. It is international in its content while seeking specially to report developments in Britain. Also included are: statistics, book reviews and letters to the editor.

British Journal of Clinical Psychology

Year of Origin: 1977
Publisher: The British Psychological Society, St. Andrews House, 48 Princess Road East, Leicester LE 1 7DR, UK. Tel: 01 44 6931
Editor: Dr. D. A. Shapiro
Subscription Rate: $85 one-year
Circulation/Frequency: 2,500/Quarterly
Pages per Issue: 100
Author Payment: None
Photo Policy: Photos Not Accepted
Scope of Journal: Publishes new findings, theoretical methodological and review papers bearing on the whole field of clinical psychology and includes: descriptive and aetiological studies of psychopathology, applications of psychology to medicine and health care, studies of assessment and treatment of psychological disorders, social and organizational aspects of psychological disorder and ill health.

British Journal of Dermatology

Publisher: Blackwell Scientific Publications Ltd., Osney Mead, Oxford OX 2 OLL
Editor: Dr. J. Burton, Dermatology Dept., Royal Infirmary, Bristol BS 2 8 HW
Subscription Rate: £50 one-year UK, £60 one-year Overseas, $135 one-year USA/Canada
Circulation/Frequency: 3,960/Monthly
Pages per Issue: 125
Author Payment: None
Photo Policy: Black and White Glossies
Writer's Guidelines: Contact Editor
Scope of Journal: This journal publishes original articles in all aspects of the normal biology, and of the pathology of the skin. The publication provides a vehicle for both experimental and clinical research and serves equally the laboratory worker and the physician.

British Journal of Haematology

Publisher: Blackwell Scientific Publications Ltd., Osney Mead, Oxford, OX 2 OEL
Editor: Dr. I. Chenarin, Dept. of Haematology, Northick Park Hospital, Clinical Research Center, Watford, Road, Harrow, Middlesex HAI 3 UJ
Subscription Rate: £66 one-year UK, £79 one-year Overseas, $187.50 one-year USA/Canada
Circulation/Frequency: 3,690/Monthly
Pages per Issue: 175
Author Payment: None
Photo Policy: Black and White Glossies
Writer's Guidelines: Contact Editor
Scope of Journal: This journal is designed to meet the needs of the practicing haematologist; publishes results of clinical and laboratory research and reviews topics of current interest.

British Journal of Medical Psychology

Year of Origin: 1977
Publisher: The British Psychological Society, St. Andrews House, 48 Princess Road East, Leicester LE 1 7DR, UK. Tel: 01 444 6931
Editor: Professor J. P. Watson
Subscription Rate: $82 one-year
Circulation/Frequency: 2,500/Quarterly
Pages per Issue: 100
Author Payment: None
Photo Policy: Photos Not Accepted
Scope of Journal: This journal publishes original papers of knowledge in the area of those aspects of psychology applicable to medicine and related clinical disciplines. Publishes articles, empirical studies, theoretical papers and clinical reports.

British Journal of Nutrition
Year of Origin: 1947
Publisher: Cambridge University
Press, 32 East 57th Street, New York,
New York 10022. Tel: 212 688 8885
Editor: Dr. R. H. Smith
Subscription Rate: $242 one-year
Circulation/Frequency:
2,392/Bimonthly
Pages per Issue: 170
Author Payment: None
Photo Policy: Black and White Glossies
Scope of Journal: This journal publishes original work in all branches of nutrition, including clinical and human nutrition including descriptions of new apparatus and techniques. The contents are subdivided into clinical and human nutrition, and general nutrition.

British Journal of Obstetrics and Gynaecology
Publisher: Blackwell Scientific Publications Ltd., 8 John Street, London
WC1N 2 E S
Editor: Dr. Frank Hytten, 27 Sussex
Place, Regents Park, London NW1
4RG
Subscription Rate: £38.50 one-year
UK, £46 one-year Overseas, $105
one-year USA
Circulation/Frequency: 1,000 per annum/12 yearly
Pages per Issue: about 4690
Author Payment: None
Photo Policy: Black and White Glossies
Writer's Guidelines: Contact Editor
Scope of Journal: This journal is aimed at both the practicing clinician and the clinical scientist; the core of the journal consists of reports of original research, clinical case reports, book reviews and a correspondence column.

The British Medical Bulletin
Publisher: Churchill Livingstone, British Council, 5 Bentinck Street, London WIMSRN. Tel: 01 935 9121
Editor: Fiona Foley
Subscription Rate: £22 one-year
Circulation/Frequency: 4,500/3 yearly
Pages per Issue: 100 average
Author Payment: £500 per paper
Photo Policy: 3 × 5 Black and White Glossies
Writer's Guidelines: Contact Editor
Scope of Journal: Publishes collections of authoritative research papers relevant to medical practitioners and research workers in the field. Each issue considers a completely different topic e.g. the 1982 issues are: Alcohol and Disease. Contributors are invited; unsolicited manuscripts are not accepted.

Bulletin of the History of Medicine
Year of Origin: 1926
Publisher: The Johns Hopkins University Press, Baltimore, Maryland
21218. Tel: 301 338 7811
Editor: Lloyd G. Stevenson
Subscription Rate: $18 one-year Individual, $31 one-year Institution
Circulation/Frequency: 3,000/Quarterly
Pages per Issue: about 144
Author Payment: None
Photo Policy: Photos Not Accepted
Writer's Guidelines: Contact Editor
Scope of Journal: The scope of this journal is designated through the title.

Canada's Mental Health
Year of Origin: 1953
Publisher: Department of National
Health and Welfare of Canada,
Health Services & Promotion Branch,
Ottawa, Canada KIA 1B4. Tel: 613
995 0166
Editor: Brenda Wattie

Subscription Rate: $5.50 one-year USA/Foreign, free in Canada
Circulation/Frequency: 32,000/Quarterly
Pages per Issue: 28–36
Author Payment: None
Photo Policy: Photos Not Accepted
Scope of Journal: This journal publishes articles, book reviews, brief reports and announcements of interest to a multidisciplinary readership in the human services field.

Canadian Journal of Public Health
Year of Origin: 1910
Publisher: Canadian Public Health Association, 1335 Carling Avenue, Suite 210, Ottawa, Ontario, KIZ 8N8. Tel: 613 725 3769
Editor: John M. Last, MD
Subscription Rate: $20 one-year Canada, $25 one-year USA, $30 one-year Foreign
Circulation/Frequency: 5,000/Bimonthly
Pages per Issue: 72
Author Payment: None
Photo Policy: Black and White Glossies
Writer's Guidelines: Contact Editor
Scope of Journal: Publishes a variety of articles and material of interest and use to health professionals and students in the public health field. The journal also contains book reviews, meeting and conference announcements, employment services, and welcomes letters to the editor.

Canadian Medical Association Journal
Year of Origin: 1911
Publisher: Canadian Medical Association, Box 8650, Ottawa, KIG 0G8, Ontario, Canada. Tel: 613 731 9331
Editor: Peter P. Morgan, MD, Scientific Editor, David Woods, Director of Publications
Subscription Rate: $60 one-year USA, $49.50 one-year Canada
Circulation/Frequency: 35,000/Bi-monthly
Pages per Issue: 150 average
Author Payment: No payment for scientific manuscripts; 22¢/word for journalistic articles
Photo Policy: Photos Not Accepted
Scope of Journal: The purpose of this journal is to keep physicians current not only in science but also with economic and practice management information to help them apply science for the benefit of their patients. As well as original and review articles, there are departments on health care delivery, conference reports and the political process. This publication attempts to keep doctors well-informed about every aspect of their professional lives.

Cancer
Year of Origin: 1901
Publisher: J. B. Lippincott Company, East Washington Square, Philadelphia, Pennsylvania 19105. Tel: 215 574 4200
Editor: Jonathan E. Rhoades, MD
Subscription Rate: $50 one-year USA Individual, $55 one-year USA Institution, $85 one-year Foreign Individual, $90 one-year Foreign Institution
Circulation/Frequency: Unavailable/24 yearly
Pages per Issue: Variable
Author Payment: None
Photo Policy: Photos Not Accepted
Writer's Guidelines: Contact Editor
Scope of Journal: A journal of the American Cancer Society, Inc. which publishes original articles covering the full range of concerns related to the diagnosis and treatment of the various forms of cancer. It covers such topics as surgical and medical treatment, pathology, statistics, education and experimental work.

Cancer Metastisis Reviews
Year of Origin: 1982
Publisher: Martinus Nijhoff, Box 566, 2501 CN The Hague, The Netherlands. Tel: 070 469 460
Editor: Isaiah J. Fidler, DVM, Ph.D., Frederick Cancer Research Center, Post Office Box B, Frederick, Maryland 21701, USA
Subscription Rate: $48 one-year Individual USA, $80 one-year Institution USA, (Airmail add $9)
Circulation/Frequency: New/Quarterly
Pages per Issue: about 80–100
Author Payment: None
Photo Policy: Photos Not Accepted
Writer's Guidelines: Contact Editor
Scope of Journal: A new review journal which aims to provide critical perspectives on new developments in this rapidly developing field. It will emphasize both basic and clinical research and include topics such as tumor progression, pathogenesis of metastasis, the metastatic phenotype, host factors, new methods for studies, and new developments in the diagnosis and treatment of metastasis.

Cancer Research
Year of Origin: 1940
Publisher: Waverly Press, Inc., 428 East Preston Street, Baltimore, Maryland 21202. Tel: 301 528 4000
Editor: Dr. Peter N. Magee, Fels Research Institute, Temple University School of Medicine, Philadelphia, Pennsylvania 19140. Tel: 215 221 4720
Subscription Rate: $80 one-year Individual, $140 one-year Institution, $40 one-year Member
Circulation/Frequency: 6,000/Monthly
Pages per Issue: 420
Author Payment: None
Photo Policy: Black and White Glossies

Scope of Journal: Publishes significant original research in the fields of cancer and cancer-related biomedical science. It also contains review articles, communications, letters to the editor, meeting reports, announcements of interest, notices of recent deaths, and a periodic lists of books received.

Cell and Tissue Kinetics
Publisher: Blackwell Scientific Publications Ltd., Osney Mead, Oxford OX 2 OLL
Editor: Prof. N. A. Wright, Department of Histopathology, Royal Postgraduate Medical School, Hammersmith Hospital, Duane Road, London W 12 OHS
Subscription Rate: £ 60 one-year UK, £ 72 one-year Overseas, $165 one-year USA
Circulation/Frequency: 810/Bimonthly
Pages per Issue: about 30
Author Payment: None
Photo Policy: Black and White Glossies
Writer's Guidelines: Contact Editor
Scope of Journal: Devoted to studies of cell proliferation and differentiation in normal and abnormal states. The journal publishes papers covered both with kinetics at the cellular level and with those aspects of molecular biology that have a bearing on cell proliferation.

Child and Adolescent Social Work Journal
Year of Origin: 1983
Publisher: Human Sciences Press, Inc., 72 Fifth Avenue, New York, New York 10011. Tel: 212 243 6783
Editor: Florence Lieberman, D.S.W.
Subscription Rate: $26 one-year Individual, $58 one-year Institution
Circulation/Frequency: New/4 yearly
Pages per Issue: 80
Author Payment: None

Photo Policy: Black and White Glossies
Writer's Guidelines: No Specific Guidelines; Use Format Within Journal
Scope of Journal: This is an informative new journal which will feature original articles focusing on clinical social work practice with children, adolescents, and their families.

Child and Family Behavior Therapy
Year of Origin: 1979
Publisher: Haworth Publishing Company, 28 East 22nd Street, New York, New York 10010. Tel: 212 228 2800
Editor: Cyril M. Franks, Applied and Prof. Psychology, Busch Campus, Rutgers University, Box 819, Piscataway, New York 08854
Subscription Rate: $36 one-year Individual, $45 one-year Institution, $75 one-year Library
Circulation/Frequency: 1,100/Quarterly
Pages per Issue: Variable
Author Payment: None
Photo Policy: Photos Not Accepted
Writer's Guidelines: Contact Editor
Scope of Journal: Research and clinical applications in behavior therapy with children and adolescents, as well as the enhancement of parenting.

Child: Care, Health and Development
Publisher: Blackwell Scientific Publications, 8 John Street, London WC1N 2ES, England.
Editor: Dr. R. B. Jones
Subscription Rate: $90 one-year USA and Canada
Circulation/Frequency: 710/6 yearly
Pages per Issue: about 80
Author Payment: None
Photo Policy: Black and White Glossies Accepted

Writer's Guidelines: Contact Editor
Scope of Journal: The aim of this journal is to promote the study of the development of all children, particularly those handicapped by physical, intellectual, emotional and social problems and to provide information on new methods to help overcome their problems.

Child Care Quarterly
Year of Origin: 1971
Publisher: Human Science Press, 72 Fifth Avenue, New York, New York 10011. 212 243 6000
Editor: Jerome Beker
Subscription Rate: $55 Institution, $23 Individual
Circulation/Frequency: 1900/Quarterly
Pages per Issue: 80 average
Author Payment: None
Photo Policy: Black and White Glossies
Writer's Guidelines: No Specific Guidelines; Use Format Within Journal
Scope of Journal: This journal is an independent professional publication committed to the improvement of child care practice in a variety of day and residential settings and to the advancement of this field. Designed to serve child care workers, their supervisors, and other personnel in child care settings as well as instructors and students in the field; this publication provides a channel of communication and debate.

Childhood Education
Year of Origin: 1924
Publisher: Association for Childhood Education, International, 3615 Wisconsin Avenue NW, Washington, D. C. 20016. Tel: 202 363 6963
Editor: Lucy Prete Martin
Subscription Rate: $23 one-year Individual, $27 one-year Institution, $20

one-year Branch, $10 one-year Student/Retired
Circulation/Frequency: 15,000/five yearly
Pages per Issue: 72
Author Payment: 100% contributed
Photo Policy: 8 × 10 Black and White Glossies
Scope of Journal: This journal is a professional medium for those concerned with the education and well-being of children from infancy through teacher educators, parents child care workers, librarians, supervisors, administrators and others.

Child Psychiatry and Human Development: An International Journal
Year of Origin: 1969
Publisher: Human Science Press, 72 Fifth Avenue, New York, New York 10011. Tel: 212 243 6000
Editor: John C. Duffy
Subscription Rate: $58 Institution, $28 Individual
Circulation/Frequency: 1,250/Quarterly
Pages per Issue: 80 average
Author Payment: None
Photo Policy: Black and White Glossies
Writer's Guidelines: No Specific Guidelines; Use Format Within Journal
Scope of Journal: The purpose of this journal is to serve allied professional groups of specialists in child psychiatry, social science, pediatrics, psychology, and human development in their task: to define the developing child and adolescent in health and in conflict. As an interdisciplinary and independent forum, it publishes articles from all points of view.

Children's Health Care
Year of Origin: 1970
Publisher: Charles B. Slack, Inc.,

6900 Grove Road, Thoeofare, New Jersey 08086. Tel: 609 848 1000
Editor: Mary C. Cerreto, PhD
Subscription Rate: $19 one-year
Circulation/Frequency: 300/Quarterly
Pages per Issue: 48 maximum
Author Payment: None
Photo Policy: Photos Not Accepted
Scope of Journal: The purpose of this publication is directed to research studies as well as essays, speeches and other efforts which foster the psychosocial care of children and families in health care settings.

Circulation
Year of Origin: 1950
Publisher: American Heart Association, 7320 Greenville Avenue, Dallas, Texas 75231. Tel: 214 750 5300
Editor: Elliot Rapaport, MD
Subscription Rate: $40 one-year USA, $55 one-year Foreign
Circulation/Frequency: 25,000/Monthly
Pages per Issue: Variable
Author Payment: None
Photo Policy: Black and White or Color. Color Cost paid by author
Scope of Journal: Devoted to research and advances in the cardiovascular field. It presents original articles, symposia, editorials, current topics, case reports, and letters to the editor.

Circulation Research
Year of Origin: 1958
Publisher: American Heart Association, 7320 Greenville Avenue, Dallas, Texas 75231. Tel: 214 750 5300
Editor: Francois M. Abboud, MD
Subscription Rate: $75 one-year USA, $90 one-year Foreign
Circulation/Frequency: 4,500/Monthly
Pages per Issue: Variable
Author Payment: None
Photo Policy: Black and White or

Color. Color Cost paid by author
Scope of Journal: This journal is concerned with basic research in the cardiovascular field. It publishes original articles and editorials for clinicians interested in basic science and for research workers in anatomy, biology, biochemistry, biophysics, microbiology, physiology, pharmacology, and pathology, as well as experimental medicine.

Clinical Allergy
Publisher: Blackwell Scientific Publications, Osney Mead, Oxford OX 2 OEL, England. Tel: 0865 40201
Editor: Dr. J. W. Kerr, Dept. of Respiratory Medicine, Glasgow G11 6NT, Scotland. Dr. W. E. Parish, Environment Safety Division, Cohworth/Wehwyn Laboratory, Cohworth House, Shanbrook, Bedford MK44 1LO
Subscription Rate: $145 one-year USA and Canada
Circulation/Frequency: 1,420/6 yearly
Pages per Issue: 100
Author Payment: None
Photo Policy: Black and White Glossies Accepted
Writer's Guidelines: Contact Editors
Scope of Journal: Publishes papers dealing with clinical and experimental observations in disease and in all fields of health care in which allergic hypersensitivity plays a part.

Clinical Endocrinology
Publisher: Blackwell Scientific Publications Ltd., 8 John Street, London SC1N 2ES
Editor: Professor L. Rees, Dr. D. T. Baird, 8 John Street, London SC1N 2ES
Subscription Rate: £90 one-year UK, £108 one-year Overseas, $255 one-year USA/Canada
Circulation/Frequency: 1,240/Monthly

Pages per Issue: about 110
Author Payment: None
Photo Policy: Black and White Glossies
Writer's Guidelines: Contact Editor
Scope of Journal: Publishes papers dealing with the human endocrine disorder, its pathogenesis, diagnosis and treatment. The purpose of the journal is to define clinical endocrinology in its widest terms and to encourage an international view of the subject by publication of papers from all parts of the world.

Clinical and Experimental Dermatology
Publisher: Blackwell Scientific Publications Ltd., Osney Mead, Oxford OX 2 0LL
Editor: Dr. M. Black, Dept. of Histopathology, Institute of Dermatology, St. John's Hospital for Diseases of the Skin, Lisle Street, London WC2H 7BJ
Subscription Rate: £62 one-year UK, £75 one-year Overseas, $172 one-year USA/Canada
Circulation/Frequency: 950/Bimonthly
Pages per Issue: about 30
Author Payment: none
Photo Policy: Black and White Glossies
Writer's Guidelines: Contact Editor
Scope of Journal: This journal publishes original articles covering all aspects of the normal biology of the skin and clinical and experimental dermatology.

Clinical and Experimental Immunology
Publisher: Blackwell Scientific Publications Ltd., 8 John Street, London SC1N 2ES
Editor: Professor J. L. Turk, 8 John Street, London SC1N 2#S
Subscription Rate: £160 one-year UK,

£192.50 one-year Overseas, $450 one-year USA/Canada
Circulation/Frequency: 1,960/Monthly
Pages per Issue: about 225
Author Payment: None
Photo Policy: Black and White Glossies
Writer's Guidelines: Contact Editor
Scope of Journal: This journal publishes original research on the role of immunology in the diagnosis and pathogenesis of disease, including allergy. The journal's wide brief includes the study of methods to control the immunological reaction, the production of disease in experimental animals by immunological reaction procedures, transplantation and cancer immunology, etc.

Clinical and Experimental Pharmacology and Physiology

Publisher: Blackwell Scientific Publications, 99 Burry Street, Carlton, Victoria 3053, Australia
Editor: M. J. Rand, A. E. Doyle, J. P. Coghlan, P. I. Korner
Subscription Rate: $205 one-year USA & Canada
Circulation/Frequency: 490/6 yearly
Pages per Issue: 100
Author Payment: None
Photo Policy: Black and White Glossies Accepted
Writer's Guidelines: Contact Editors
Scope of Journal: This journal provides a medium for the rapid publication of original research papers and short communications on the results of work in pharmacology and physiology, and includes critical comments together with replies by the original author of papers which appeared in earlier issues.

Clinical Gerontologist

Year of Origin: 1982
Publisher: Haworth Publishing Company, 28 East 22nd Street, New York, New York 10010. Tel: 212 228 2800
Editor: T. L. Brink, Palo Alto School of Prof. Psych., 467 Hamilton Avenue, Palo Alto, California 94301
Subscription Rate: $24 one-year Individual, $60 one-year Institution, $75 one-year Library
Circulation/Frequency: Unavailable/Quarterly
Pages per Issue: Variable
Author Payment: None
Photo Policy: Photos Not Accepted
Writer's Guidelines: Contact Editor
Scope of Journal: This is a journal of aging and mental health presenting timely material relevant to the needs of mental health professionals; practitioners who deal with aged clients.

Clinical Nuclear Medicine

Year of Origin: 1976
Publisher: J. B. Lippincott Company, East Washington Square, Philadelphia, Pennsylvania 19105. Tel: 215 574 4216
Editor: Sheldon Baum, M. D., Milton S. Hershey Medical Center, Hershey, Pennsylvania 17033
Subscription Rate: $39 one-year USA, $48 one-year Foreign
Circulation/Frequency: 3026/Monthly
Pages per Issue: about 45
Author Payment: None
Photo Policy: Black and White Glossies
Scope of Journal: This journal welcomes the submission of material related to the clinical aspects of nuclear medicine. Emphasis is on scanning, imaging and related subjects.

Clinical Orthopaedics and Related Research

Year of Origin: 1953
Publisher: J. B. Lippincott Company, East Washington Square, Philadelphia, Pennsylvania 19105. Tel: 215 574 4200
Editor: Dr. Marshall R. Urist
Subscription Rate: $98 one-year
Circulation/Frequency: Unavailable/10 yearly
Pages per Issue: Variable
Author Payment: None
Photo Policy, Photos Not Accepted
Writer's Guidelines: Contact Publisher
Scope of Journal: Original articles describing investigations, advances, or observations related to the title of this journal.

Clinical Otolaryngology

Publisher: Blackwell Scientific Publications Ltd., 8 John Street, London SC1N 2ES
Subscription Rate: £50 one-year UK, £60 one-year Overseas, $135 one-year USA/Canada
Circulation/Frequency: 860/Bi-monthly
Pages per Issue: about 20
Author Payment: none
Photo Policy: Black and White Glossies
Writer's Guidelines: Contact Editor
Scope of Journal: The journal is devoted to clinically-oriented research papers on current practice including audiology, speech pathology, head and neck plastic and reconstructive surgery and related specialties.

Clinical Pediatrics

Year of Origin: 1962
Publisher: J. B. Lippincott Company, East Washington Square, Philadelphia, Pennsylvania 19105. Tel: 215 574 4216
Editor: David Cornfeld, Editor-in-Chief, Benjamin K. Silverman, Co-editor
Subscription Rate: $35 one-year USA, $44 one-year Canada/Foreign
Circulation/Frequency: 23,220/Monthly
Pages per Issue: 50–70
Author Payment: None
Photo Policy: Black and White Glossies
Scope of Journal: This journal is practice-oriented. Manuscripts are solicited of value to the practitioner in all areas of child care. Articles may be on any topic in the area of pediatric practice, clinical research, behavioral and educational problems, community health situations, subspeciality applications and other features falling within these general realms.

Clinical Pharmacology and Therapeutics

Year of Origin: 1960
Publisher: The C. V. Mosby Company, 11830 Westline Industrial Drive, St. Louis, Missouri 83141. Tel: 314 872 8370
Editor: Walter Modell, MD, Cornell University Medical College, Box 119, Larchmont, New York, 10538
Subscription Rate: $66 one-year Institution USA, $77.50 International, $45 one-year Individual USA, $56.50 International, $36 one-year Student USA, $47.50 International
Circulation/Frequency: 6,392/Monthly
Pages per Issue: 145
Author Payment: None; Unsolicited articles subject to page charge.
Photo Policy: Black and White Glossies
Scope of Journal: The official journal of: American Society for Pharmacology and Experimental Therapeutics, American Society of Clinical Pharmacology and Therapeutics. The articles submitted for publication should

represent original communications and be submitted exclusively to this journal.

Clinical Physiology

Publisher: Blackwell Scientific Publications Ltd., 8 John Street, London WC1N 2ES

Editor: J. Wahren, Dept. Clinical Physiology, Huddinge University Hospital, S-141 86 Stockholm, Sweden

Subscription Rate: £60 one-year UK, £72 one-year overseas, $180 one-year USA/Canada

Circulation/Frequency: 500/Bimonthly

Pages per Issue: about 25

Author Payment: None

Photo Policy: Black and White Glossies

Writer's Guidelines: Contact Editor

Scope of Journal: The journal provides original reports on clinical and experimental research related to the human physiology and disease.

Clinical Preventive Dentistry

Year of Origin: 1979

Publisher: J. B. Lippincott Company, East Washington Square, Philadelphia, Pennsylvania 19105. Tel: 215 574 4216

Editor: J. H. Manhold, D.M.D., Clinical Preventive Dentistry, 352 Shunpike Road, Chatham Township, New Jersey 07928

Subscription Rate: $25 one-year Individual USA, $25 one-year Foreign, $15 one-year Student USA

Circulation/Frequency: 29,343/Bi-monthly

Pages per Issue: about 50

Author Payment: None

Photo Policy: Black and White Glossies

Scope of Journal: This journal is designed for publication of research papers and other articles of highest quality relevant to the practitioner concerned with prevention and control of oral disease.

Clinical Reproduction and Fertility

Year of Origin: 1982

Publisher: Blackwell Scientific Publications, 99 Burry Street, Carlton, Victoria 3053, Australia

Editor: W. Jones

Subscription Rate: $125 one-year USA & Canada

Circulation/Frequency: Unavailable/Quarterly

Pages per Issue: Variable

Author Payment: None

Photo Policy: Black and White Glossies Accepted

Writer's Guidelines: Contact Editor

Scope of Journal: Research on human reproduction and fertility especially aspects of infertility.

Clinics in Chest Medicine

Year of Origin: 1980

Publisher: W. B. Saunders, West Washington Square, Philadelphia, Pennsylvania 19105. Tel: 215 574 4700

Editor: Guest Editor for Each Issue

Subscription Rate: $26 one-year

Circulation/Frequency: Unavailable/3 yearly

Pages per Issue: about 250

Author Payment: None

Photo Policy: Black and White Glossies

Scope of Journal: Hard cover periodical. Each issue is focused on a specific topic and contains 10 to 15 state-of-the-art reviews on current clinical practice by leading specialists in the field. Unsolicited articles are not accepted. The "guest editor" of each issue invites papers on the areas of current interest.

Clinics in Endocrinology and Metabolism

Year of Origin: 1972
Publisher: W. B. Saunders, 1 St. Anne's Road, Eastbourne, East Sussex BN21 3, United Kingdom. Tel: USA 215 574 4700
Editor: Guest Editor For Each Issue
Subscription Rate: $48 one-year
Circulation/Frequency: Unavailable/3 yearly
Pages per Issue: about 250
Author Payment: None
Photo Policy: Black and White Glossies
Scope of Journal: Hard cover periodical. Each issue is focused on a specific topic and contains 10 to 15 state-of-the-art reviews on current clinical practice by leading specialists in the field. Unsolicited articles are not accepted. The "guest editor" of each issue invites papers on areas of current interest.

Clinics in Gastroenterology

Year of Origin: 1972
Publisher: W. B. Saunders, 1 St. Anne's Road, Eastbourne, East Sussex BN21 3, United Kingdom. Tel: USA 215 574 4700
Editor: Guest Editor For Each Issue
Subscription Rate: $48 one-year
Circulation/Frequency: Unavailable/3 yearly
Pages per Issue: about 250
Author Payment: None
Photo Policy: Black and White Glossies
Scope of Journal: Hard cover periodical. Each issue is focused on a specific topic and contains 10 to 15 state-of-the-art reviews on current clinical practice by leading specialists in the field. Unsolicited articles are not accepted. The "guest editor" of each issue invites papers on areas of current interest.

Clinics in Haematology

Year of Origin: 1972
Publisher: W. B. Saunders, West Washington Square, Philadelphia, Pennsylvania 19105. Tel: 215 574 4700
Editor: Guest Editor For Each Issue
Subscription Rate: $48 one-year
Circulation/Frequency: Unavailable/3 yearly
Pages per Issue: about 250
Author Payment: None
Photo Policy: Black and White Glossies
Scope of Journal: Hard cover periodical. Each issue is focused on a specific topic and contains 10 to 15 state-of-the-art reviews on current clinical practice by leading specialists in the field. Unsolicited articles are not accepted. The "guest editor" of each issue invites papers on areas of current interest.

Clinics in Immunology and Allergy

Year of Origin: 1981
Publisher: W. B. Saunders, 1 St. Anne's Road, Eastbourne, East Sussex BN 21 3, United Kingdom. Tel: USA 215 574 4700
Editor: Guest Editor For Each Issue
Subscription Rate: $48 one-year
Circulation/Frequency: Unavailable/3 yearly
Pages per Issue: about 250
Author Payment: None
Photo Policy: Black and White Glossies
Scope of Journal: Hard cover periodical. Each issue is focused on a specific topic and contains 10 to 15 state-of-the-art reviews on current clinical practice by leading specialists in the field. Unsolicited articles are not accepted. The "guest editor" of each issue invites papers on areas of current interest.

Clinics in Laboratory Medicine
Year of Origin: 1981
Publisher: W. B. Saunders, West Washington Square, Philadelphia, Pennsylvania 19105. Tel: 215 574 4700
Editor: Guest Editor For Each Issue
Subscription Rate: $30 one year
Circulation/Frequency: Unavailable/3 yearly
Pages per Issue: about 250
Author Payment: None
Photo Policy: Black and White Glossies
Scope of Journal: Hard cover periodical. Each issue is focused on a specific topic and contains 10 to 15 state-of-the-art reviews on current clinical practice by leading specialists in the field. Unsolicited articles are not accepted. The "guest editor" of each issue invites papers on areas of current interest.

Clinics in Obstetrics and Gynaecology
Year of Origin: 1974
Publisher: W. B. Saunders, 1 St. Anne's Road, Eastbourne, East Sussex BN 21 3, United Kingdom. Tel: USA 215 574 4700
Editor: Guest Editor For Each Issue
Subscription Rate: $48 one-year
Circulation/Frequency: Unavailable/3 yearly
Pages per Issue: about 250
Author Payment: None
Photo Policy: Black and White Glossies
Scope of Journal: Hard cover periodical. Each issue is focused on a specific topic and contains 10 to 15 state-of-the-art reviews on current clinical practice by leading specialists in the field. Unsolicited articles are not accepted. The "guest editor" of each issue invites papers on areas of current interest.

Clinics in Perinatology
Year of Origin: 1974
Publisher: W. B. Saunders, West Washington Square, Philadelphia, Pennsylvania 19105. Tel: 215 574 4700
Editor: Guest Editor For Each Issue
Subscription Rate: $30 one-year
Circulation/Frequency: Unavailable/3 yearly
Pages per Issue: about 250
Author Payment: None
Photo Policy: Black and White Glossies
Scope of Journal: Hard cover periodical. Each issue is focused on a specific topic and contains 10 to 15 state-of-the-art reviews on current clinical practice by leading specialists in the field. Unsolicited articles are not accepted. The "guest editor" of each issue invites papers on areas of current interest.

Clinics of Plastic Surgery
Year of Origin: 1974
Publisher: W. B. Saunders, West Washington Square, Philadelphia, Pennsylvania 19105. Tel: 215 574 4700
Editor: Guest Editor For Each Issue
Subscription Rate: $60 one-year
Circulation/Frequency: Unavailable/Quarterly
Pages per Issue: about 250
Author Payment: None
Photo Policy: Black and White Glossies
Scope of Journal: Hard cover periodical. Each issue is focused on a specific topic and contains 10 to 15 state-of-the-art reviews on current clinical practice by leading specialists in the field. Unsolicited articles are not accepted. The "guest editor" of each issue invites papers on areas of current interest.

Clinics in Rheumatic Diseases
Year of Origin: 1975
Publisher: W. B. Saunders, 1 St.
Anne's Road, Eastbourne, East Sussex
BN 21 3, United Kingdom. Tel: USA
215 574 4700
Editor: Guest Editor For Each Issue
Subscription Rate: $48 one-year
Circulation/Frequency: Unavailable/3
yearly
Pages per Issue: about 250
Author Payment: None
Photo Policy: Black and White Glossies
Scope of Journal: Hard cover periodical. Each issue is focused on a
specific topic and contains 10 to 15
state-of-the-art reviews on current
clinical practice by leading specialists
in the field. Unsolicited articles are
not accepted. The "guest editor" of
each issue invites papers on areas of
current interest.

Clinics in Sports Medicine
Year of Origin: 1982
Publisher: W. B. Saunders, West
Washington Square, Philadelphia,
Pennsylvania 19105. Tel: 215 574
4700
Editor: Guest Editor For Each Issue
Subscription Rate: $30 one-year
Circulation/Frequency: Unavailable/3
yearly
Pages per Issue: about 250
Author Payment: None
Photo Policy: Black and White Glossies
Scope of Journal: Hard cover periodical. Each issue is focused on a
specific topic and contains 10 to 15
state-of-the-art reviews on current
clinical practice by leading specialists
in the field. Unsolicited articles are
not accepted. The "guest editor" of
each issue invites papers on areas of
current interest.

Community Mental Health Journal
Year of Origin: 1963
Publisher: Human Science Press, 72
Fifth Avenue, New York, New York
10011. Tel: 212 243 6000
Editor: Allen Beigel, Herbert Diamond
Subscription Rate: $58 Institution,
$28 Individual
Circulation/Frequency: 3,400/Quarterly
Pages per Issue: 96 average
Author Payment: None
Photo Policy: Black and White Glossies
Writer's Guidelines: No Specific
Guidelines; Use Format Within Journal
Scope of Journal: This publication is
the only periodical devoted
specifically to coordinate emergent
approaches to mental health and social well-being. Among subjects covered are crisis intervention, planned
change, suicide prevention, social system analysis, early case finding, family therapy, milieu therapy, human
ecology, high-risk groups, and social
welfare programs.

Contemporary Education Review
Year of Origin: 1981
Publisher: American Educational Research Association, 1230 17th Street,
NW, Washington, D. C. 20036. Tel:
202 223 9485
Editor: Dr. Frank Farley, University
of Wisconsin, Madison, Wisconsin
53703
Subscription Rate: $14 one-year Individual, $17 one-year Institution, $12
one-year Members
Circulation/Frequency: 1982 estimate
2,000/Quarterly
Pages per Issue: 80
Author Payment: None
Photo Policy: Photos Not Accepted
Scope of Journal: Publishes scholarly

reviews of books, including monographs, learning and instructional materials and products, media and nonprint educational products and educational technology products related to educational issues.

Contemporary Psychology
Year of Origin: 1956
Publisher: American Psychological Association, 1200 17th Street, NW, Washington, D. C. 20036. Tel: 202 833 7686
Editor: Donald J. Foss, Dept. of Psychology, University of Texas at Austin, Austin, Texas 78712
Subscription Rate: $15 one year member, $40 one year nonmember
Circulation/Frequency: 7,500/Monthly
Pages per Issue: 1
Author Payment: None
Photo Policy: Black and White Glossies
Scope of Journal: Contains critical reviews of books, films, tapes, and other media relevant to psychology.

Critical Care Quarterly
Year of Origin: 1978
Publisher: Aspen Systems Corporation, 1600 Research Blvd, Rockville, Maryland 20850. Tel: 301 251 5000
Editor: John Marozsan
Subscription Rate: $38 one-year
Circulation/Frequency: 7,000/Quarterly
Pages per Issue: 96–100
Author Payment: None
Photo Policy: Black and White Glossies
Scope of Journal: This journal publishes articles geared toward nurses, paramedics, and associated health care providers in the critical care area.

Culture, Medicine and Psychiatry
Year of Origin: 1977
Publisher: Department of Psychiatry and Behavior Sciences, University of Washington, School of Medicine, Seattle, Washington 98195, USA
Editor: D. Reidel, Box 17, 3300 AA Dordrecht, Holland
Subscription Rate: $55 USA Institution, $21 USA Individual
Circulation/Frequency: 1,000/Quarterly
Pages per Issue: 100
Author Payment: None
Photo Policy: Photos Not Accepted
Scope of Journal: This journal serves as an international and interdisciplinary forum for three interrelated fields: medical and psychiatric anthropology; cross-cultural psychiatry; and related cross-societal clinical and epidemiological studies. It publishes original research, theoretical papers, and review articles on all subjects in each of these fields.

CURATIONIS—The South African Journal of Nursing
Publisher: South African Nursing Association, Box 1280, Pretoria, 0001 R. S.A. Tel: 44-3306
Editor: Frieda Paton
Subscription Rate: $12 one-year USA
Circulation/Frequency: 2,000/Quarterly
Pages per Issue: 56
Author Payment: None
Photo Policy: Photos Not Accepted
Scope of Journal: This journal publishes scientific articles on all aspects of nursing; includes book reviews as well as summaries of completed nursing research in South Africa.

Current Surgery
Year of Origin: 1933
Publisher: J. B. Lippincott Company, East Washington Square, Philadel-

phia, Pennsylvania 19105. Tel: 215 574 4216
Editor: Lloyd M. Nyhus, M. D., University of Illinois at the Medical Center, Box 6998, Chicago, Illinois 60680
Subscription Rate: $28 one-year USA, $34 one-year Foreign
Circulation/Frequency: 2,549/Bi-monthly
Pages per Issue: about 40
Author Payment: None
Photo Policy: Black and White Glossies (Colored at Author's Expense)
Scope of Journal: This journal is designed for the publication of current abstracts of the world's surgical literature. In addition, original articles will be published which relate to the following aspects of surgery: (1) Review; (2) Current concepts; (3) History; and (4) Preliminary reports of original research (clinical or experimental).

Dairy Council Digest
Year of Origin: 1927
Publisher: National Dairy Council, 6300 North River Road, Rosemont, Illinois 60018. Tel: 312 696 1020
Editor: Lois Mc Bean, 1654 Morehead Drive, Ann Arbor, Michigan 48103. Tel: 313 667 3512
Subscription Rate: $18 one-year
Circulation/Frequency: 76,400/6 yearly
Pages per Issue: 6–10
Author Payment: None
Photo Policy: Photos Not Accepted
Writer's Guidelines: Contact Editor; No Unsolicited Articles
Scope of Journal: This Digest is an interpretive review of recent nutrition research information for professional people. Emphasis is placed on subjects relating to food, nutrition, health and the importance of a well-balanced diet. There are also brief abstracts of selected published nutrition information.

Dental Abstracts
Year of Origin: 1955
Publisher: American Dental Association, 211 East Chicago Avenue, Chicago, Illinois 60611. Tel: 312 440 2782
Editor: Kate Spencer
Subscription Rate: $24 one-year USA, $32 one-year Foreign
Circulation/Frequency: 7,500/Monthly
Pages per Issue: 56
Author Payment: None
Photo Policy: Photos Not Accepted
Scope of Journal: Abstracts related to dentistry and other health-related fields.

Dental Clinics of North America
Year of Origin: 1956
Publisher: W. B. Saunders, West Washington Square, Philadelphia, Pennsylvania 19105. Tel: 215 574 4700
Editor: Guest Editor For Each Issue
Subscription Rate: $30 one-year
Circulation/Frequency: Unavailable/Bi-monthly
Pages per Issue: about 250
Author Payment: None
Photo Policy: Black and White Glossies
Scope of Journal: Hard cover periodical. Each issue is focused on a specific topic and contains 10 to 15 state-of-the-art reviews on current clinical practice by leading specialists in the field. Unsolicited articles are not accepted. The "guest editor" of each issue invites papers on areas of current interest.

Dental Hygiene
Year of Origin: 1927
Publisher: American Dental Hygienists' Association, 444 North Michigan Avenue, Chicago, Illinois 60611. Tel: 312 440 8920
Editor: Jan Seefeldt

Subscription Rate: $40 one-year, $75 two-years, $110 three-years, $4 single copy
Circulation/Frequency: 30,000/Monthly
Pages per Issue: 48
Author Payment: None
Photo Policy: Black and White Glossies & Color
Scope of Journal: This journal includes scientific, research, and feature articles for the benefit of ADHA members and other health professionals.

Dimensions in Health Science
Year of Origin: 1924
Publisher: Canadian Hospital Association, CHA 8th Floor 410 Laurier Ave. West Ottawa, Ontario, Canada, KIR 7T6. Tel: 613 238 8005
Editor: Carol Wightman
Subscription Rate: Variable
Circulation/Frequency: 13,000/Monthly
Pages per Issue: 48
Author Payment: 85% contributed; $100 per published page
Photo Policy: Black and White Glossies
Scope of Journal: This is a journal for health care professionals; topics include: cost control, management, health law, technology, and specific "how-to" articles about different hospital issues.

Directory of On-Going Research in Smoking and Health
Year of Origin: 1966
Publisher: Department of Health and Human Services, 5600 Fishers Lane (Park 158), Public Health Service, Rockville, Maryland 20857. Tel: 301 443 1690
Editor: Donald R. Shopland
Subscription Rate: free
Circulation/Frequency: 7,000/every other year
Pages per Issue: 439
Author Payment: None
Photo Policy: Photos Not Accepted
Writer's Guidelines: Contact Editor
Scope of Journal: A subject and name (plus affiliation) index of international research programs focusing on smoking and its health hazards.

Diseases of the Colon & Rectum
Year of Origin: 1958
Publisher: J. B. Lippincott Company, East Washington Square, Philadelphia, Pennsylvania 19105. Tel: 215 574 4216
Editor: John R. Hill, M.D., 403 First National Bank Bldg., Rochester, Minnesota 55901
Subscription Rate: $60 one-year USA, $72 one-year Canada/Foreign
Circulation/Frequency: 4,230/Monthly
Pages per Issue: 60–80
Author Payment: None
Photo Policy: Black and White Glossies up to 5 × 7
Scope of Journal: This journal is designed for the publication of original papers that constitute significant contributions to the advancement of knowledge within the special field designated by the name of this journal.

Drug Information Journal
Year of Origin: 1977
Publisher: Drug Information Association, Medical Documentation Service, 19 South 22nd Street, Philadelphia, Pennsylvania 19103. Tel: 1 215 563 1238
Editor: Alberta D. Berton
Subscription Rate: $25
Circulation/Frequency: 1,500/Quarterly
Pages per Issue: about 400
Author Payment: None

Photo Policy: Black and White Glossies

Scope of Journal: A variety of topics are considered for publication in this journal, such as: the new drug approval process, regulations and their effect on the drug development process, directives for preparation of new drug applications, advertising prescription drugs, the drug registration process, drug regulatory affairs, causal relationships between drugs and their adverse effects, etc.

Educational Evaluation and Policy Analysis

Year of Origin: 1979
Publisher: American Educational Research Association, 1230 17th Street NW, Washington, D. C. 20036. Tel: 202 223 9485
Editor: Dr. Eva Baker, UCLA, Los Angeles, California 90052
Subscription Rate: $16 one-year Individual, $21 one-year Institution, $12 one-year Member
Circulation/Frequency: 3,100/Quarterly
Pages per Issue: 128
Author Payment: None
Photo Policy: Camera Ready Accepted
Scope of Journal: Focuses on educational evaluation, educational policy analysis, and the relationship between the two activities. It strives to serve the multiple needs of the diverse specialists currently working in educational evaluation. It deals not only with theoretical and methodological issues, but also with the intensely practical concerns of individuals engaged in the evaluation enterprises and the formulation of educational policy.

Educational Researcher

Year of Origin: 1972
Publisher: American Educational Research Association, 1230 17th Street, N. W., Washington, D. C. 20036.
Tel: 202 223 9485
Editor: Dr. William Russell
Subscription Rate: $14 one-year Individual, $17 one-year Institution
Circulation/Frequency: 14,000/10 yearly
Pages per Issue: 32
Author Payment: None
Photo Policy: Black and White Half Tones Accepted
Scope of Journal: Contains scholarly articles of general significance to the educational research and development community from a wide range of disciplines. It is also designed to report current research, news, government policies, and to serve as the forum for the membership.

Educational Technology

Year of Origin: 1961
Publisher: Educational Technology Publications, Inc., 140 Sylvan Avenue, Englewood Cliffs, New Jersey 07643.
Tel: 201-871-4007
Editor: Lawrence Lipsitz
Subscription Rate: $49 Domestic, $59 Foreign
Circulation/Frequency: 5,000/Monthly
Pages per Issue: 64
Author Payment: None
Photo Policy: Black and White Glossies
Scope of Journal: This journal is the world's leading periodical covering the fields of educational media and technology, including computer usage for education and training, all forms of audio-visual communication, and the systematic design of instruction. Articles range from theoretical to practical applications; emphasis on technology as applied science.

Readers in more than one hundred countries.

Education Week
Year of Origin: 1983
Publisher: Editorial Projects in Education, Suite 560, 1333 New Hampshire Avenue, NW, Washington D. C. 20036. Tel: 202 466 5190
Editor: Ron Wolk
Subscription Rate: $39.94 one-year
Circulation/Frequency: Unavailable/Weekly
Pages per Issue: 24 pages
Author Payment: None
Photo Policy: Photos Not Accepted
Writer's Guidelines: Follow Format in Journal
Scope of Journal: This newsletter is for the entire education community which serves as a common forum where colleagues in private and public education can share ideas and opinions regularly. In short, this publication records the saga of American education—court decisions, government actions, commission reports, research results, what goes on in the classroom, and the ongoing human story of the people who make it work and make it worthwhile.

Emergency Health Services Quarterly
Year of Origin: 1980
Publisher: Haworth Publishing Company, 28 East 22nd Street, New York, New York 10010. Tel: 212 228 2800
Editor: Ralph D'Agostino, Dept. of Cardiology, Boston City Hospital, Sears Bldg. Room 108, 818 Harrison Avenue, Boston, Massachusetts 02118
Subscription Rate: $48 one-year Individual, $60 one-year Institution, $75 one-year Library
Circulation/Frequency: 2,775/Quarterly

Pages per Issue: Variable
Author Payment: None
Photo Policy: Photos Not Accepted
Writer's Guidelines: Contact Editor
Scope of Journal: This journal provides a forum for thoughtful discussion of the major planning, operation, and research issues facing emergency medical services.

Emergency Medical Abstracts
Year of Origin: 1978
Publisher: Charles B. Slack, Inc., 6900 Grove Road, Thorofare, New Jersey 08086. Tel: 609 848 1000
Editor: W. Richard Bukata, MC
Subscription Rate: $85 one-year
Circulation/Frequency: 1,100/Monthly
Pages per Issue: 20–25
Author Payment: None
Photo Policy: Photos Not Accepted
Writer's Guidelines: Not Applicable
Scope of Journal: This publication provides abstracts of current literature in Emergency Medicine, and to promote exchange of new ideas among Emergency Medicine specialists through a convenient reprint exchange system.

Emergency Medicine
Year of Origin: 1969
Publisher: Steve Fischer, 280 Madison Avenue, New York, New York 10016. Tel: 212 889 4530
Editor: Douglas W. E. Wagner
Subscription Rate: $32.50 one-year USA, $25.00 one-year Physicians, $21.00 one-year Students, $45.00 one-year Foreign
Circulation/Frequency: 133,000/23 yearly
Pages per Issue: Variable
Author Payment: None
Photo Policy: Photos Not Accepted
Scope of Journal: Articles present immediately usable information on the diagnosis and treatment of common

emergencies and on the acute phases of other illnesses and injuries.

Environment

Year of Origin: 1958
Publisher: Heldref Publishing Company, 4000 Albemarle Street, NW, Washington, D. C. 20016. Tel: 202 362 6445
Editor: Jane Scully
Subscription Rate: $15 one-year Individual, $20 one-year Institution, $5 add for foreign, $2 add for newsstand
Circulation/Frequency: 15,000/10 per year
Pages per Issue: 45
Author Payment: Most are contributed; Others $75–$100 by length
Photo Policy: Black and White 3 × 5 and larger; Transparencies
Scope of Journal: The purpose of this journal is to provide insights from the natural and social sciences and technology into issues which affect the physical, biological, or social environment. The journal presents facts and analyses in a manner which usefully informs public decision-making. Articles are published which report original research or interpret the results of research. The editor encourages well-founded discussions of controversial policy issues.

Environmental Health Perspectives

Year of Origin: 1972
Publisher: National Institute of Environmental Health Sciences, Box 12233, Research Triangle Park, North Carolina 27709. Tel: 919 541 3406
Editor: Gary E. R. Hook, George W. Lucier
Subscription Rate: $41 one-year USA, $51.25 one-year Foreign, $7 single issue USA, $8.75 single issue Foreign
Circulation/Frequency:
2,500/Bi-monthly
Pages per Issue: 240
Author Payment: None
Photo Policy: Black and White Glossies
Scope of Journal: The objective of this journal is to communicate research findings of environmental health significance and to inform the scientific community of potential health hazards that are associated with particular elements in the environment. It publishes conference and workshop proceedings, perspective statements on selected problem areas, toxicologic information summaries, overviews of areas on environmental health, and reviews on specific problems and agents. Unsolicited manuscripts are also published.

Family and Child Mental Health Journal

Year of Origin: 1975
Publisher: Human Science Press, 72 Fifth Avenue, New York, New York 10011. Tel: 212 243 6000
Editor: Paul Pressman
Subscription Rate: $36 Institution, $16 Individual
Circulation/Frequency: 1,700/Bi-annual
Pages per Issue: 96 average
Author Payment: None
Photo Policy: Black and White Glossies
Writer's Guidelines: No Specific Guidelines; Use Format Within Journal
Scope of Journal: This journal serves an important function for the professional community by providing an interdisciplinary approach to family and child therapy. To promote understanding and effective clinical practice, families and children must be viewed in a social and psychological context. An eclectic forum of psy-

chologists, psychiatrists, social workers, educators, and sociologists illustrates the field's most significant theoretical and therapeutic advances.

Family and Community Health
Year of Origin: 1978
Publisher: Aspen Systems Corporation, 1600 Research Blvd. Rockville, Maryland 20850. Tel: 301 251 5000
Editor: Adina Reinhardt, Ph.D.
Subscription Rate: $49.25
Circulation/Frequency: 2,500/Quarterly
Pages per Issue: 100
Author Payment: None
Photo Policy: 3 × 5 Black and White Glossies
Scope of Journal: The approach in this journal is holistic with an emphasis on health promotion and maintenance. Each issue focuses on a specific predetermined topic pertinent to family and community health.

Family Life Educator
Year of Origin: 1982
Publisher: National Family Life Education Network, ETR Associates, 1700 Mission Street, Suite 203, Santa Cruz, California 95060. Tel: 408 429 9822
Editor: Mary Nelson
Subscription Rate: Membership $20 one-year (which includes Journal)
Circulation/Frequency: 4,000/4 yearly
Pages per Issue: about 40
Author Payment: None
Photo Policy: Black and White Glossies
Writer's Guidelines: Follow Format in Journal
Scope of Journal: This quarterly will provide the subscriber with up-to-date information and practical teaching techniques to help insure the continuing quality of your educational efforts. It will provide information on programs, people, and issues throughout the U. S. including: teaching ideas, informational summaries, law and public policy, religious perspectives, items for parents, reproducible articles and handouts and book, film, and journal reviews.

Family Planning Perspectives
Year of Origin: 1969
Publisher: The Alan Guttmacher Institute, 360 Park Avenue, New York, New York 10010. Tel: 212 685 5858
Editor: Richard Lincoln
Subscription Rate: $18.50 one-year, $9.25 one-year/$30 membership
Circulation/Frequency: 24,200/Bi-monthly
Pages per Issue: 48–64
Author Payment: None
Photo Policy: Black and White Glossies
Scope of Journal: This journal publishes original research in the field of family planning/population, as well as reports of meetings, research and development in the field. The focus is on family planning programs, reproductive research, contraceptive technology, biomedical research, evaluation of programs, policy analysis, fertility trends, abortion, contraceptive practice and relevant legal analysis. Book reviews, special reports and comments are also published.

Family Practice Research Journal
Year of Origin: 1980
Publisher: Human Sciences Press, Inc., 72 Fifth Avenue, New York, New York 10011. Tel: 212 243 6783
Editor: Jack M. Stack, M.D.
Subscription Rate: $28 one-year Individual, $74 one-year Institution
Circulation/Frequency: 488/4 yearly
Pages per Issue: 64
Author Payment: None
Photo Policy: Black and White Glossies

Writer's Guidelines: No Specific Guidelines; Use Format Within Journal

Scope of Journal: This journal provides a forum for significant experimental, historical, basic, and clinical case studies. While incorporating theoretical developments in other medical specialties, the Journal addresses the unique problems and emerging treatment modalities of particular interest to family physicians and other health professionals.

Family Relations (Previously *The Family Coordinator*)
Year of Origin: 1953
Publisher: National Council on Family Relations, 1219 University Avenue SE, Minneapolis, Minnesota 55414
Editor: Michael J. Sporakowski, Virginia Tech University, 201 Wallace Hull Annex, Blacksburg, Virginia 24061. Tel: 804 961 6251
Subscription Rate: $23.50 one-year Individual, $30 one-year Institution
Circulation/Frequency: 7,000/Quarterly
Pages per Issue: 148
Author Payment: No payment to authors; Authors submit $10 processing fee
Photo Policy: Photos Not Accepted
Writer's Guidelines: Contact Editor
Scope of Journal: This journal is designed for practitioners in fields related to family and child development. Examples of topics covered: family life education, marital and family therapy, human sexuality, parent-child relationships, aging families, family violence, family stress; also includes book and media reviews.

Family Therapy
Year of Origin: 1966
Publisher: Libra Publishing Company, 391 Willets Road, Roslyn Heights,
New York 11577. Tel: 516 484 4950
Editor: Martin Blinder, M. D.
Subscription Rate: $30 Institution, $25 Individual
Circulation/Frequency: 1,000/Three Per Year
Pages per Issue: 128
Author Payment: Free Subscription
Photo Policy: Black and White Glossies or clear originals
Writer's Guidelines: American Psychological Association Style Manual
Scope of Journal: This Bulletin is devoted to the practice of family, group and other interactional therapies. A variety of directions with different treatment approaches and techniques are called for-depending on an assessment of the most effective way of proceeding. The articles selected reflect this multi-faceted approach.

Family Therapy News
Year of Origin: 1942
Publisher: American Association for Marriage and Family Therapy, 924 West 9th Street, Upland, California 91786
Editor: William J. Hiebert, S. T. M.
Subscription Rate: $10 one year
Circulation/Frequency: 10,000/Bimonthly
Pages per Issue: 16
Author Payment: None
Photo Policy: Photos Not Accepted
Writer's Guidelines: Contact Publisher
Scope of Journal: *The Family Therapy News* offers broad coverage of recent news developments in the field of marriage and family therapy.

Hastings Center Report
Year of Origin: 1971
Publisher: Institute of Society, Ethics and the Life Sciences, 360 Broadway, Hastings-on-Hudson, New York 10706. Tel: 914 478 0500
Editor: Carol Levine

Subscriptiton Rate: $35 Institution, $23 Individual, $19 Student
Circulation/Frequency: 9,500/Bimonthly
Pages per Issue: 48
Author Payment: None
Photo Policy: Photos Not Accepted
Writer's Guidelines: No formal guidelines; must be typed double-spaced and accompanied by a self-addressed, stamped envelope.
Scope of Journal: Ethical issues in health care, sciences, social and behavioral sciences, and professions.

Health Care Management Review
Year of Origin: 1976
Publisher: Aspen Systems Corporation, 1600 Research Blvd., Rockville, Maryland 20850. Tel. 301 2521 5000
Editor: John R. Marozsan
Subscription Rate: $49 one-year
Circulation/Frequency: 5,000/Quarterly
Pages per Issue: 100
Author Payment: None
Photo Policy: Black and White Glossies
Scope of Journal: Publishes articles on key issues in Health Care Administration and Policy.

Health Education, Previously: School Health Review
Year of Origin: 1969
Publisher: American Alliance for Health, Physical Education, Recreation and Dance, 1900 Association Drive, Reston, Virginia 22091. Tel: 703 476 3479
Editor: Elizabeth France
Subscription Rate: $42 one-year membership, $25 Graduate Students, $22.50 Undergraduate Students. Membership dues include subscription
Circulation/Frequency: Bi-monthly
Pages per Issue: 48–64
Author Payment: None

Photo Policy: Black and White glossies any size; include photo credit and release
Scope of Journal: This is a peer-reviewed professional journal. It publishes articles on topics of relevance to health educators. Articles can be theoretical, practical, technical, philosophical, historical or controversial. Regular columns cover teaching ideas, research abstracts, history and philosophy, book reviews, new books, news and resources. Publishes special features in three issues a year.

Health Education Journal
Publisher: The Health Education Council, 78 New Oxford Street, London SC 1A 1AH, United Kingdom. Tel: 01 637 1881
Editor: Freddie Lawrence
Subscription Rate: £3 one-year
Circulation/Frequency: 4,500/Quarterly
Pages per Issue: 32–36
Author Payment: None
Photo Policy: Black and White Glossies
Writer's Guidelines: Contact Editor
Scope of Journal: This journal reflects research and developments in health education practice and theory. Papers range from general surveys to reports on specific projects. There are: news items, book reviews and opinion features.

Health Education Quarterly
Year of Origin: 1973
Publisher: Human Sciences Press, Inc., 72 Fifth Avenue, New York, New York, 10011. Tel: 212 243 6783
Editor: Marshall H. Becker, Ph.D., M.P.H., Noreen M. Clark, Ph.D., Associate Editor
Subscription Rate: $28 one-year Individual, $69 one-year Institution
Circulation/Frequency: 1675/4 yearly

Pages per Issue: 96
Author Payment: None
Photo Policy: Black and White Glossies
Writer's Guidelines: No Specific Guidelines; Use Format Within Journal
Scope of Journal: An informative journal which examines the promotion of public health through elevating the quality of health education, improving medical practices, and stimulating research. Topics of practical and theoretical importance are presented, including: alcohol and drug education, ethical issues in public health policy; the relation of health education; ethical issues in public health policy; the federal policy; occupational health education for the elderly. An invaluable journal for health care providers, and public health educators, administrators & policy-makers.

The Health Educator: A Practical Forum for Health Professionals
Year of Origin: 1983
Publisher: Krames Communications, 345-G Serramonte Plaza, Daly City, California 94015. Tel: 415 994 1150
Editor: Christine S. Kradjian, R.N., Editor-in-Chief
Subscription Rate: $17 one-year
Circulation/Frequency: Unavailable/4 yearly
Pages per Issue: 4–6
Author Payment: None
Photo Policy: Photos Not Accepted
Writer's Guidelines: No Unsolicited Articles
Scope of Journal: Programs and resources that work . . . with contact persons; how to set up a network of resources; how to build support inside and outside an organization; how to set up programs; how to find funding; how to get materials; practi-cal "hands-on" approaches and information; based on what successful programs use nationwide from hospitals, physicians' offices, industry, outpatient clinics, etc.

Health Policy Quarterly
Year of Origin: 1981
Publisher: Human Science Press, 72 Fifth Avenue, New York, New York 10011. Tel: 212 243 6000
Editor: Herbert C. Schulberg, Edmund Ricci
Subscription Rate: $74 Institution, $30 Individual
Circulation/Frequency: 1,140/Quarterly
Pages per Issue: 64 average
Author Payment: None
Photo Policy: Black and White Glossies
Writer's Guidelines: No Specific Guidelines; Use Format Within Journal
Scope of Journal: This journal stimulates vital communication between program evaluators and policymakers in all phases of public health administration. It includes the five major stages of successful service delivery: health policy formulation, program planning, experiments in health care delivery, evaluation of current health programs, and the dissemination and utilization of evaluation studies.

Health Values
Year of Origin: 1976
Publisher: Charles B. Slack, Inc., 6900 Grove Road, Thorofare, New Jersey 08086. Tel: 609 848 1000
Editor: Elizabeth A. Nielson, Ed.D., Robert C. Drake, Managing Editor
Subscription Rate: $20 one-year Individual, $25 one-year Institution
Circulation/Frequency: 2,134/Bimonthly
Pages per Issue: 40–48

Author Payment: None
Photo Policy: Black and White Glossies
Scope of Journal: This journal publishes original articles dealing with the health problems in the community and how these concerns can be remedied . . . as well as how people in the community can achieve high level wellness through proper health education and preventive care.

Heart and Lung: The Journal of Critical Care
Year of Origin: 1972
Publisher: C. V. Mosby Company, 11830 Westline Drive, St. Louis, Missouri 63141. Tel: 314 872 8370
Editor: Kathleen Dracup, RN, MN, CCRN, Sylvan Lee Weinberg, M.D., *Communication to be sent to:* Dr. Weinberg, 33 West First Street, Dayton, Ohio 45402. Tel: 513 278 2612, ext. 4215 or 3317
Subscription Rate: $15 one-year Individual USA, $36 one-year Institution USA, $12 one-year Students USA, $22 one-year Individual Foreign, $43 one-year Institution Foreign, $19 one-year Student Foreign
Circulation/Frequency: 60,000/Bi-monthly
Pages per Issue: about 110
Author Payment: None
Photo Policy: Black and White Glossies
Scope of Journal: Original articles describing investigation, advances, or observations regarding care of the critically ill patient are invited.

Home Health Care Services Quarterly
Year of Origin: 1978
Publisher: The Haworth Press, Inc., 28 East 22nd Street, New York, New York 10010. Tel: 212 228 2800
Editor: Laura Reif, RN, PhD, Dept. of Family Health Care Nursing, University of California, San Francisco, California, 94143
Subscription Rate: $32 Individual, $48 Institution, $65 Library
Circulation/Frequency: Unavailable/Quarterly
Pages per Issue: Variable
Author Payment: None
Photo Policy: Photos Not Accepted
Writer's Guidelines: Contact Editor
Scope of Journal: This journal is aimed to home health care administrators as well as gerontologists involved with the provision, evaluation, and enhancement of home health care services and related services.

Hospital and Community Psychiatry
Year of Origin: 1950
Publisher: American Psychiatric Association, 1700 18th Street, NW, Washington, D. C. 20009. Tel: 202 682 6070
Editor: John A. Talbott, MD
Subscription rate: $24 one-year
Circulation/Frequency: 18,000/Monthly
Pages per Issue: 72–80
Author Payment: None
Photo Policy: Photos Not Accepted
Scope of Journal: This is an interdisciplinary journal and is directed to professional staff members of mental health facilities and agencies. It publishes clinical and research papers, evaluative studies, review articles, commentary, and reports on legal and judicial issues and other matters of current interest or controversy— also publishes reports of unusual cases, a question-and-answer section, columns on law and psychiatry and other topical concerns; reviews of books and a calendar of meetings.

Hospital Forum
Year of Origin: 1970
Publisher: Kathryn E. Johnson, 830 Market Street, San Francisco, California 94102
Editor: Susan J. Anthony
Subscription Rate: $20 one-year
Circulation/Frequency: 12,500/Bimonthly
Pages per Issue: 50–60
Author Payment: None
Photo Policy: 5 × 7 Black and White Glossies
Writer's Guidelines: Contact Editor
Scope of Journal: Articles present innovative ideas in hospital management and are a source of practical working information.

Hospital Pharmacy
Year of Origin: 1966
Publisher: J. B. Lippincott Company, East Washington Square, Philadelphia, Pennsylvania 19105. Tel: 215 574 4216
Editor: Neil M. Davis, Hospital Pharmacy, 1143 Wright Drive, Huntingdon Valley, Pennsylvania 19006
Subscription Rate: $27 one-year USA, $34 one-year Canada/Foreign, $17 one-year Student USA
Circulation/Frequency: 24,210/Monthly
Pages per Issue: about 50
Author Payment: None
Photo Policy: Black and White Glossies
Scope of Journal: This journal welcomes manuscripts on all areas of interest to pharmacists serving inpatients and out-patients in hospitals, long-term care facilities, and other institutional settings. Submission of new information on well-publicized subjects is welcomed. Thorough documentation is required.

Hospital Progress
Year of Origin: 1920
Publisher: The Catholic Health Association of the United States, 4455 Woodson Road, St. Louis, Missouri 63134. Tel: 314 427 2500
Editor: Carol S. Boyer
Subscription Rate: $25 one-year
Circulation/Frequency: 14,000/Monthly
Pages per Issue: 100
Author Payment: None
Photo Policy: Black and White Glossies
Scope of Journal: Health care administration and management articles; also, ethical and medical-moral issues.

Hospitals
Year of Origin: 1936
Publisher: American Hospital Publishing Company, Inv., Suite 700, 211 East Chicago Avenue, Chicago, Illinois 60611
Editor: Dan Schechter
Subscription Rate: $35 one-year
Circulation/Frequency: 90,000/24 yearly
Pages per Issue: 140 average
Author Payment: Negotiated
Photo Policy: Negotiated
Scope of Journal: Articles deal with the broad issues that confront the health care field. The two most common approaches are views of a single individual and the views of several individuals put together by a writer. The subject in all cases is some issue that affects the management of health care. Case studies are also welcome, but must be short.

Hospital Topics
Year of Origin: 1922
Publisher: Hospital Topics, Inc., Box 5976, Sarasota, Florida 34277. Tel: 813 371 0188
Editor: Gordon M. Marshall

Subscription Rate: $25 one-year
Circulation/Frequency:
7,000/Bi-monthly
Pages per Issue: 48
Author Payment: None
Photo Policy: Black and White Glossies
Writer's Guidelines: Contact Editor
Scope of Journal: This journal specializes in "how-to-do-it" short illustrated articles for the busy hospital manager; there is also a question and answer column for central service, infection control, pharmacy and financial management.

Human Ecology
Year of Origin: 1973
Publisher: Plenum Publishing Company, 233 Spring Street, New York, New York 10013. Tel: 212 620 8466
Editor: Susan Lees
Subscription Rate: $72 USA, $81 Foreign
Circulation/Frequency:
Unavailable/Quarterly
Pages per Issue: 100
Author Payment: None
Photo Policy: Photos Not Accepted
Scope of Journal: This journal publishes an array of articles, materials and announcements pertinent to students and professionals in social as well as environmental sciences. Articles range from theoretical to actual case studies; contains book reviews.

Human Relations
Year of Origin: 1948
Publisher: Plenum Publishing Company, 233 Spring Street, New York, New York 10013. Tel: 212 620 8466
Editor: Michael Foster
Subscription Rate: $130
Circulation/Frequency:
Unavailable/Monthly
Pages per Issue: 100
Author Payment: None

Photo Policy: Photos Not Accepted
Scope of Journal: This journal publishes an array of articles, materials, and announcements pertinent to students and professionals in all social sciences. Articles range from theoretical to actual case studies.

Hypertension
Year of Origin: 1979
Publisher: American Heart Association, 7320 Greenville Avenue, Dallas, Texas 75231. Tel: 214 750 5300
Editor: Harriet P. Dunstan, MD
Subscription Rate: $40 one year USA, $55 one-year Foreign
Circulation/Frequency: 3,000/6 yearly
Pages per Issue: Variable
Author Payment: None
Photo Policy: Black and White or Color, Color Cost paid by author
Scope of Journal: Reports clinical and laboratory investigation in hypertension. The entire field of hypertension is covered through reports of original investigations, brief reveiws, symposia and case reports. Designed for anyone interested in hypertension.

Imagination, Cognition and Personality
Year of Origin: 1981
Publisher: Baywood Publishing Company, 120 Marine Street, P.O. Box D, Farmingdale, New York, 11735. Tel: 516 249 2464
Editor: Kenneth S. Pope, Jerome L. Singer, Yale University, Box 11A, Yale Station, New Haven, Connecticut 06520
Subscription Rate: $55 Institution, $30 Individual
Circulation/Frequency: 500/Quarterly
Pages per Issue: about 96
Author Payment: Lead Author Receives Complimentary Copies of Issue + 20 Free Reprints

Photo Policy: Black and White Glossies
Scope of Journal: This journal presents thoughtful explorations of the flow of images, fantasies, memory fragments and anticipations, which constitute our moment-to-moment experience of awareness.

Immunology
Publisher: Blackwell Scientific Publications Ltd., 8 John Street, London SC1N 2ES
Editor: L. E. Glynn, MRC Rheumaticism, Research Unit, Canadian Red Cross Memorial Hospital, Taplow, Maidenhead, Berkshire, England
Subscription Rate: £107.50 one-year UK, £129 one-year overseas, $295 one-year USA/Canada
Circulation/Frequency: 2,520/Monthly
Pages per Issue: about 100
Author Payment: None
Photo Poloicy: Black and White Glossies
Writer's Guidelines: Contact Editor
Scope of Journal: Publishes papers describing original work in all areas of immunology including cellular immunology, immunochemistry, immunogenetics, allergy, transplantation immunology, cancer immunology and clinical immunology.

Imprint
Year of Origin: 1968
Publisher: National Student Nurses Association, 10 Columbus Circle, New York, New York 10009. Tel: 212 581 2211
Editor: Full-time nursing student elected annually
Subscription Rate: $8 one-year, 15 two-years, 22 three-years
Circulation/Frequency: 35,000/5 yearly
Pages per Issue: 76–96
Author Payment: None
Photo Policy: Black and White Glossies 5 × 7 or 8 × 10
Scope of Journal: This journal publishes articles that are not purely personal accounts or fiction but generally rely on the literature. Ideas and interpretations attributed to another person, or facts discovered by another writer, must be documented.

Infection and Immunity
Year of Origin: 1970
Publisher: American Society for Microbiology, 1913 I Street, NW, Washington, D. C. 20006. Tel: 202 833 9680
Editor: J. W. Shands, Jr.
Subscription Rate: $120 one-year
Circulation/Frequency: 7,086/Monthly
Pages per Issue: 1,266
Author Payment: Author Pays $20 per published page, May Request To Waive Charges
Photo Policy: Photos Not Accepted
Scope of Journal: This journal accepts manuscripts covering all aspects of the pathogenesis of infection including model infections by bacteria, fungi, and unicellular parasites; viral infections; and immune methanisms. Oral microbiology and immunology are given extensive coverage.

International Health News
Year of Origin: 1982
Publisher: National Council for International Health, 2121 Virginia Avenue, NW, Suite 303, Washington, D. C. 20037. Tel: 202 298 5901
Editor: Virgil E. McMahan
Subscription Rate: $25 one-year with membership
Circulation/Frequency: 6,500/Bimonthly
Pages per Issue: 12–16
Author Payment: 100% Contributed
Photo Policy: 3 × 5 Black and White Glossies
Writer's Guidelines: Contact Editor

Scope of Journal: Contains news and special features to keep professionals and students informed of international health activities. The emphasis is on timely topics and innovative programs of both public and private sector agencies and organizations with regular columns on such topics as educational opportunities, new publications and audiovisuals, workshop and conference schedules, and legislative updates.

The International Journal of Aging and Human Development

Year of Origin: 1970
Publisher: Baywood Publishing Company, Inc., 120 Marine Street, Box D, Farmingdale, New York 11735. Tel: 516 249 2464
Editor: Robert J. Kastenbaum, 1149 East Vinedo Lane, Tempe, Arizona 85281
Subscription Rate: $45 one-year Individual, $76 one-year Institution
Circulation/Frequency: 2,000/8 yearly
Pages per Issue: 96 average
Author Payment: Complimentary Copy to lead author plus 20 free reprints
Photo Policy: Black and White glossies
Scope of Journal: Trend-setting reports, critical reviews, case histories, and essays represent the very latest research in intergenerational relations, institutionalizations, work and retirements, social action, and many other vital issues. Rigorous peer-reviews by an editorial board of national and international experts insures the highest standards of scholarship.

International Journal of Epidemiology

Publisher: Oxford University Pres, St. Thomas Hospital Medical School, London SE 1 7 EH, England. Tel: 01 928 9292
Editor: C. du V Florey
Subscription Rate: $65 one-year
Circulation/Frequency: 2,100/Quarterly
Pages per Issue: 96
Author Payment: None
Photo Policy: Photos Not Accepted
Scope of Journal: Manuscripts include: original work, reviews and letters to the editor in the fields of research and teaching epidemiology.

International Journal of Health Services

Year of Origin: 1970
Publisher: Baywood Publishing Company, Inc., 120 Marine Street, Farmingdale, New York, 11735. Tel: 516 293 7130
Editor: Vicente Navarro
Subscription Rate: $25 Individual, $55 Institution, $20 Student, $4 Postage Outside USA
Circulation/Frequency: 2,000/Quarterly
Pages per Issue: 175–225
Author Payment: 100% Contributed; Complimentary Copies to Author
Photo Policy: Black and White Glossies
Scope of Journal: This journal analyzes what is going on in the health profession. It analyzes different forces that shape the nature of health, disease, medicine and public health in our societies. It covers subjects of health policy, social policy; health economics; political economy; sociology, history and philosophy; and ethics and law. It is open to all points of view and gives priority to positions that are underrepresented in current debates.

International Journal of Family Therapy

Year of Origin: 1962
Publisher: Human Sciences Press, 72 Fifth Avenue, New York, New York 10011. Tel: 212 243 6000
Editor: Gerald H. Zuk
Subscription Rate: $56 Institution, $25 Individual
Circulation/Frequency: 1,300/Quarterly
Pages per Issue: 64–80
Author Payment: None
Photo Policy: Black and White Glossies
Writer's Guidelines: No Specific Guidelines; Use Format Within Journal
Scope of Journal: This journal presents the latest developments in theory, research, and practice with an emphasis on examining the family within the socioeconomic matrix of which it is an integral part. Essential factors which are examined include family value systems, social class, racial, religious, and ethnic background. Also included are significant cross-cultural and transnational studies with implications for all those concerned with this growing field.

International Journal of Law and Psychiatry

Year of Origin: 1977
Publisher: The Pergamon Press, Maxwell House, Fairview Park, Elsford, New York 10523. Tel: 913 592 7700
Editor: David N. Weisstib
Subscription Rate: $75 one-year
Circulation/Frequency: 1,000/Quarterly
Pages per Issue: 120 average
Author Payment: None
Photo Policy: Photos Not Accepted
Scope of Journal: This journal is intended to provide a multidisciplinary forum for the exchange of ideas and information among professionals concerned with the interface of law and psychiatry. The journal seeks to enhance understanding and cooperation in the field through the varied approaches represented not only by law and psychiatry but also by the social sciences and related disciplines.

International Journal of Mental Health

Year of Origin: 1972
Publisher: M. E. Sharpe, Inc., 80 Business Park Drive, Armonk, New York, 10504. Tel: 914 273 1800
Editor: Arnold C. Tovell
Subscription Rate: $119 Institution, $39 Individual
Circulation/Frequency: International/Quarterly
Pages per Issue: 100
Author Payment: None
Photo Policy: Photos Not Accepted
Scope of Journal: Original articles devoted to current developments in mental health research, clinical practice and systems of care. Book reviews are accepted.

The International Journal of Psychiatry in Medicine

Year of Origin: 1970
Publisher: Baywood Publishing Company, 120 Marine Street, Box D, Farmingdale, New York 11735. Tel: 516 249 2464
Editor: Donald R. Sweeney. MD, PhD, Fair Oaks Hospital, Summit, New Jersey 07901
Subscription Rate: $51 Institution, $25 Individual
Circulation/Frequency: 1200/Quarterly
Pages per Issue: about 96
Author Payment: Lead Author Receives Complimentary Copies of Issue + 20 Free Reprints
Photo Policy: Black and White Glossies

Scope of Journal: This journal is committed to research carried out within the increasingly broad conceptual framework to which the term "psychosomatic" is applicable. It publishes articles which apply the methods of psychiatry and psychology to the further understanding of disorders which are not primarily psychiatric.

International Journal of Social Psychiatry

Year of Origin: 1955
Publisher: The International Journal of Social Psychiatry, 140 Harley Street, London, W 1 1 AH, England. Tel: 01 455 2922
Editor: Dr. Joshua Bierer
Subscription Rate: $25 one-year USA Individual, $50 one-year USA Institution
Circulation/Frequency: Unavailable/Quarterly
Pages per Issue: 80
Author Payment: None
Photo Policy: Photos Not Accepted
Scope of Journal: Manuscripts considered of interest to all professionals working in the fields of Mental Health, Research, Education.

International Journal of Systematic Bacteriology

Year of Origin: 1951
Publisher: American Society for Microbiology, 1913 I Street, NW, Washington, D. C. 20006. Tel: 202 833 9680
Editor: Erwin F. Lessel
Subscription Rate: $15 one-year Individual, $36 one-year Institution
Circulation/Frequency: 2,309/Quarterly
Pages Per Issue: 268
Author Payment: None unless articles exceed 50 printed pages
Photo Policy: Photos Not Accepted

Scope of Journal: This is the official journal of the International Committee on Systematic Bacteriology of the International Union of Microbiological Societies. It publishes papers concerned with the systematics of bacteria, yeasts, and yeastlike organisms.

International Nursing Review

Publisher: International Council of Nurses, P.O. Box 42, CH-1211 Geneva 20, Switzerland. Tel: (002) 33-64-00
Editor: Ms Merren Tardivelle
Subscription Rate: $20 USA
Circulation/Frequency: 3,000/6 yearly
Pages Per Issue: 32
Author Payment: None; one complimentary copy of issue and 50 reprints
Photo Policy: Black and White Glossies
Scope of Journal: Nursing and health affairs worldwide; programs of the International Council of Nurses and its 95 national member associations around the world; reports of international nursing and health meetings.

The International Quarterly: Community Health Education

Year of Origin: 1970
Publisher: Baywood Publishing Company, Inc., 120 Marine Street, Box D, Farmingdale, New York 11735. Tel: 516 249 2464
Editor: George P. Cernada, University of Massachusetts, Amherst, Massachusetts
Subscription Rate: $25 one-year Individual, $45 one-year Institution (add $3 postage USA/Canada and $7 postage elsewhere)
Circulation/Frequency: 500 /4 yearly
Pages per Issue: 85
Author Payment: Lead Author Receives Complimentary Copies of Issue

+ 20 Free Reprints

Photo Policy: Black and White Glossies

Scope of Journal: This new journal deals with health education and its relationship to social change. Stimulating case studies, policy reviews, and applied research written to meet the needs of health educators, program planners, behavioral scientists, policy specialists, consumer activists and related social and health professionals. Emphasis on combining maximum readability with scholarly standards and suggesting environmental and structural changes as alternatives to victim blaming strategies.

Investigative Ophthalmology and Visual Science

Year of Origin: 1962

Publisher: The C. V. Mosby Company, 11830 Westline Industrial Drive, St. Louis, Missouri 63141. Tel: 314 872 8370

Editor: Alan M. Laties, MD, 51 North 39th Street, Philadelphia, Pennsylvania 19104. Tel: 215 662 8692

Subscription Rate: $77 one-year Institution USA, $89 International, $56 one-year Individual USA, $68 International, $44.80 one-year Student USA, $56.80 International

Circulation/Frequency: 3,904/Monthly

Pages per Issue: 140

Author Payment: None

Photo Policy: Black and White Glossies

Scope of Journal: This journal is the official publication of Association for Research in Vision and Ophthalmology. Articles submitted for publication should represent original communications related to this title and submitted exclusively to this journel.

Investigative Radiology

Year of Origin: 1966

Publisher: J. B. Lippincott Company, East Washington Square, Philadelphia, Pennsylvania 19105. Tel: 215 574 4216

Editor: Richard H. Greenspan, M. D., Yale University School of Medicine, Department of Diagnostic Radiology, 333 Cedar Street, New Haven, Connecticut 06510

Subscription Rate: $50 one-year Individual USA, $54 one-year Institution USA, $60 one-year Individual Foreign, $64 one-year Institution Foreign

Circulation/Frequency: 2,059/Bimonthly

Pages per Issue: 60–80

Author Payment: None

Photo Policy: Black and White Glossies

Scope of Journal: This journal is devoted to the early publication of well-formulated original reports of investigations in diagnostic radiology, the diagnostic use of radio-active isotopes, ultrasound, infrared thermography, and related modalities. Also include reviews of articles of significance which appear in other journals; letters to the editors; review articles, summarizing topics of current investigative interest.

The Jamaican Nurse

Year of Origin: 1961

Publisher: The Nurses Association of Jamaica, 4 Trevgninon Pk Rd, KGN 5

Editor: S. Marshall Burnett

Subscription Rate: $15 one-year USA

Circulation/Frequency: International/Quarterly

Pages per Issue: 40–45

Author Payment: 25% contributed and solicited articles

Photo Policy: Photos Not Accepted

Writer's Guidelines: Contact Editor
Scope of Journal: This journal is the official publication of the Nurses Association of Jamaica. It contains professional scientific articles, news, and reports of interest to nurses and other health professionals.

The Journal of Allergy and Clinical Immunology

Year of Origin: 1929
Publisher: C. V. Mosby Company, 11830 Westline Industrial Drive, St. Louis, Missouri 63141. Tel: 314 872 8370
Editor: Charles E. Reed, MD, Journal Office West 15B Mayo Building, 200 First Street SW, Rochester, Minnesota 55901. Tel: 507 284 8675
Subscription Rate: $53.50 one-year Institution USA, $66.50 one-year International, $32.50 one-year Individual USA, $45.50 one-year International, $26.00 one-year Students USA, $39.00 one-year International
Circulation/Frequency: 7,675/Monthly
Pages per Issue: 110
Author Payment: None
Photo Policy: Black and White Glossies
Scope of Journal: This journal is directed to the needs of the clinical allergist, also reaches progressive dermatologists, internists, general practitioners, pediatricians concerned with the manifestations of allergies. It serves as the official journal of The American Academy of Allergy.

Journal of the American Academy of Dermatology

Year of Origin: 1979
Publisher: The C. V. Mosby Company, 11830 Westline Industrial Drive, St. Louis, Missouri 63141. Tel: 314 872 8370
Editor: J. Graham Smith, Jr. MD,

Medical College of Georgia, Augusta, Georgia 30912. Tel: 404 828 4684
Subscription Rate: $53 one-year Institution USA, $68.25 International, $32 one-year Individual USA, $47.25 International, $24 one-year Student USA, $39.25 International
Circulation/Frequency: 8.824/Monthly
Pages per Issue: 110
Author Payment: None
Photo Policy: Black and White Glossies
Scope of Journal: The official journal of American Academy of Dermatology and articles submitted for publication should represent original communications related to the title submitted exclusively to this journal.

Journal of the American College Health Association

Year of Origin: 1953
Publisher: American College Health Association, 152 Rollins Avenue, Suite 208, Rockville, Maryland 20852. Tel: 301 468 6868
Editor: James B. Mc Clenahan, MD
Subscription Rate: $30 one-year USA, $33 one-year Foreign
Circulation/Frequency: Unavailable/Bimonthly
Pages per Issue: 45–50
Author Payment: None
Photo Policy: Photos Not Accepted
Writer's Guidelines: Contact Editor
Scope of Journal: This journal is dedicated to the presentation of material of interest to those charged with responsibility for health programs in institutions of higher education. Topics include: Student Health Services, Mental Health Needs of Students, Action for a Better Environment, Tuberculosis Control in Colleges, etc.

The Journal of the American Dental Association

Year of Origin: 1913
Publisher: American Dental Association, 211 East Chicago Avenue, Chicago, Illinois 60611. Tel: 312 440 2782
Editor: Roger Scholle, DDS
Subscription Rate: $20 one-year USA, $32 one-year Foreign
Circulation/Frequency: 130,000/Monthly
Pages per Issue: 170
Author Payment: None
Photo Policy: Photos Not Accepted
Scope of Journal: This journal invites submission of articles, clinical reports, brief reports, reviews, perspectives, practice management, and conference summaries pertinent to dentistry, education and other health-related fields. Articles are accepted for publication with the understanding they have not been published elsewhere.

Journal of the American Dietetic Association

Year of Origin: 1923
Publisher: The American Dietetic Association, 430 North Michigan, Chicago, Illinois 60611. Tel: 312 280 5016
Editor: Dorothea F. Turner, RD
Subscription Rate: $27.50 one-year with membership
Circulation/Frequency: 54,000/Monthly
Pages per Issue: 100–180
Author Payment: 100% contributed
Photo Policy: 8 × 10 Black and White Glossies
Scope of Journal: This journal publishes refereed reports of original research and other papers covering the broad aspects of dietetics, including nutrition and diet therapy, community nutrition, education and training, and administration.

Journal of American Geriatrics Society

Year of Origin: 1953
Publisher: W. B. Saunders Company, West Washington Square, Philadelphia, Pennsylvania 19105. Tel: 215 574 4874
Editor: Paul B. Beeson, MD
Subscription Rate: $40 one-year Individual, $50 one-year Institution (add $10 foreign/$30 air)
Circulation/Frequency: 9,000/Monthly
Pages per Issue: 64
Author Payment: None
Photo Policy: Photos Not Accepted
Scope of Journal: This journal is the official publication of the American Geriatrics Society; it is dedicated to the presentation of high quality original articles reporting latest clinical findings in the fields of geriatric medicine and gerontology; also included are papers, reports, editorials, book reviews, and letters to the editor.

Journal of the American Medical Association

Year of Origin: 1848
Publisher: American Medical Association, 535 North Dearborn, Chicago, Illinois 60610. Tel: 312 751 6079
Editor: George D. Lundberg, MD
Subscription Rate: $36 one-year
Circulation/Frequency: 265,000/Weekly
Pages per Issue: 100
Author Payment: None
Photo Policy: Black and White Glossies Accepted
Scope of Journal: This journal publishes current research and clinical studies in medicine.

Journal of Andrology
Year of Origin: 1980
Publisher: J. B. Lippincott Company, East Washington Square, Philadelphia, Pennsylvania 19105. Tel: 215 574 4216
Editor: Andrezj Bartke, Ph.D., University of Texas Health Sciences Center, 7703 Floyd Curl Drive, San Antonio, Texas 78284. Tel: 512 691 6677
Subscription Rate: $49 one-year USA, $57 one-year Foreign
Circulation/Frequency: 689/Bi-monthly
Pages per Issue: 60–80
Author Payment: None
Photo Policy: Black and White Glossies
Scope of Journal: This journal publishes original papers and reviews on clinical and laboratory research pertinent to structure and function of the male reproductive system and male gametes. Except for abstracts of papers presented to the annual meeting of the ASA, the journal does not publish material that will be published elsewhere.

Journal of Applied Bacteriology
Year of Origin:
Publisher: Blackwell Scientific Publications Ltd., 8 John Street, London SC1N 2ES
Editor: C. H. Collins, 8 John Street, London SC1N 2ES
Subscription Rate: £58 one-year UK, £72 one-year overseas, $165 one-year USA/Canada
Circulation/Frequency: 3,500/Bimonthly
Pages per Issue: about 55
Author Payment: None
Photo Policy: Black and White Glossies
Writer's Guidelines: Contact Editor
Scope of Journal: The purpose of this journal is to further the study of microbiology in its application to industries.

Journal of Applied Behavioral Science
Year of Origin: 1965
Publisher: Herbert Johnson JAI Press, Inc., 36 Sherwood Place, Greenwich, Connecticut 06830. Tel: 203 629 1662
Editor: Louis A. Zurcher, Box 9155, Rosslyn Station, Arlington, Virginia 22209
Subscription Rate: $40 Institution, $33 Individual
Circulation/Frequency: 3,500/Quarterly
Pages per Issue: 144
Author Payment: None
Photo Policy: Photos Not Accepted
Scope of Journal: Publishes articles on theories of planned change applicable to individuals and systems, strategies of social intervention or innovation, the interplay among theory, practice, and values in the domain of planned change.

Journal of Applied Behavior Analysis
Year of Origin: 1967
Publisher: Department of Psychology, State University of New York, Albany, New York 12222. Tel: 518 457 3300
Editor: David Barlow
Subscription Rate: $22 one-year
Circulation/Frequency: 6,500/Quarterly
Pages per Issue: 200
Author Payment: None
Photo Policy: Photos Not Accepted
Writer's Guidelines: Contact Editor
Scope of Journal: This journal is primarily for the original publication of reports of experimental research involving applications of the experimental analysis of behavior to prob-

lems of social importance. It will also publish technical articles relevant to such research and discussion of issues arising from behavioral applications.

Journal of Applied Physiology: Respiratory, Environmental and Exercise Physiology
Year of Origin: 1887
Publisher: American Physiological Society, 9650 Rockville Pike, Bethesda, Maryland 20014. Tel: 301 530 7160
Editor: Stephen R. Geiger
Subscription Rate: $115 USA, $135 Foreign
Circulation/Frequency: Unavailable/Monthly
Pages per Issue: about 500
Author payment: None
Photo Policy: Black and White Glossies
Scope of Journal: Publishes original papers that deal with normal or abnormal function in five discrete, but often related, areas: Respiratory Physiology, Nonrespiratory function of the lungs, Environmental physiology, Exercise physiology, Interdependence.

Journal of Applied Psychology
Year of Origin: 1917
Publisher: American Psychological Association, 1200 17th Street, NW, Washington, D. C. 20036. Tel: 202 833 7686
Editor: Robert M. Guion, Dept. of Psychology, Bowling Green State University, Bowling Green, Ohio 43403
Subscription Rate: $19 one-year member, $38 one-year nonmember
Circulation/Frequency: 6,600/Bimonthly
Pages per Issue: 7–8
Author Payment: None
Photo Policy: Black and White Glossies
Scope of Journal: Devoted primarily

to original investigations that contribute new knowledge and understanding to any field of applied psychology except clinical psychology. Of interest are psychologists doing work in universities, industry, government, urban affairs, police and correctional systems, health and educational institutions, transportation and defense systems, and consumer affairs.

Journal of Bacteriology
Year of Origin: 1951
Publisher: American Society for Microbiology, 1913 I Street, NW, Washington, D. C. 20006. Tel: 202 833 9680
Editor: Simon Silver
Subscription Rate: $190 one-year
Circulation/Frequency: 8,518/Monthly
Pages per Issue: 1,495
Author Payment: Authors Pay $25 per published page. May Request To Waive Charges
Photo Policy: Photos Not Accepted
Scope of Journal: This journal is a leading periodical worldwide. It is devoted to the advancement and dissemination of fundamental knowledge concerning bacterial and other microorganisms.

Journal of Behavioral Medicine
Year of Origin: 1978
Publisher: Plenum Publishing Company, 233 Spring Street, New York, New York 10013. Tel: 212 620 8466
Editor: Dr. W. Doyle Gentry
Subscription Rate: $52 USA, $59 Foreign
Circulation/Frequency: Unavailable/Quarterly
Pages per Issue: 100
Author Payment: None
Photo Policy: Photos Not Accepted
Scope of Journal: This journal publishes an array of articles, materials and announcements pertinent to stu-

dents and professionals in the behavioral sciences, and medicine. Articles range from theoretical to case studies.

Journal of Behavior Therapy and Experimental Psychiatry
Year of Origin: 1970
Publisher: Pergamon Press, Maxwell House, Fairview Park, Elmsford, New York 10523. Tel: 914 592 7700
Editor: Joseph Wolpe, M.D., Temple University Medical School, Philadelphia, Pennsylvania 19129
Subscription Rate: $120 one-year
Circulation/Frequency: 3,500/Quarterly
Pages per Issue: 408
Author Payment: None
Photo Policy: Photos Not Accepted
Scope of Journal: This journal publishes original papers in the fields indicated by its title. One of its aims is to bring behavior therapy squarely into the domain of the psychiatrist. Besides presenting original work, the journal publishes material intended to help overcome the training gap in behavior therapy for the medically trained therapist. It includes descriptions of therapeutic methods, case reports and transcriptions of interviews.

Journal of Bioethics
Year of Origin: 1981
Publisher: Human Science Press, 72 Fifth Avenue, New York, New York 10011. Tel: 212 243 6000
Editor: Jane A. Boyajian Raible
Subscription Rate: $62 Institution, $28 Individual
Circulation/Frequency: 800/Bi-annual
Pages per Issue: 64 average
Author Payment: None
Photo Policy: Black and White Glossies
Writer's Guidelines: No Specific Guidelines; Use Format Within Journal

Scope of Journal: This periodical offers an invaluable opportunity for the open discussion of biomedical advances and concurrent social concerns which are directly related to the practice of medicine, research goals, health policies, and current legislative and judicial trends. A journal for professionals and laypersons to critically assess these complex health, policy, and moral issues.

Journal of Child Psychology and Psychiatry
Year of Origin: 1959
Publisher: The Pergamon Press, Maxwell House, Fairview Park, Elmsford, New York 10523. Tel: 914 592 7700
Editor: Dr. L. A. Hersov, Consultant Psychiatrist, Children & Adolescent's Dept., The Maudsley Hospital, London, England SE 58A7
Subscription Rate: $90 one-year
Circulation/Frequency: 3,000/Quarterly
Pages per Issue: 200
Author Payment: None
Photo Policy: Photos Not Accepted
Scope of Journal: This journal is primarily concerned with child psychology and child psychiatry including experimental and developmental studies, especially developmental psychopathology. It is recognized that many other disciplines have an important contribution to make in furthering knowledge of the mental life and behavior of children and contributions from these areas are welcome.

Journal of Chronic Diseases
Year of Origin: 1947
Publisher: The Pergamon Press, Maxwell House, Fairview Park, Elmsford, New York 10523. Tel: 914 592 7700
Editor: David P. Earle
Subscription Rate: $195 one-year

Circulation/Frequency: 3,000/Monthly
Pages per Issue: 30–40 average
Author Payment: None
Photo Policy: Photos Not Accepted
Scope of Journal: This journal is concerned with research in chronic illness, and in the domain, sometimes called Clinical Epidemiology, that is formed by the interplay of clinical medicine, epidemiology, and biostatistics. The research can be oriented toward methods, content, or both.

Journal of Clinical Psychology
Year of Origin: 1945
Publisher: Clinical Psychology Publishing Co., Inc., 4 Conant Square, Brandon, Vermont 05733. Tel: 802 247 6871
Editor: Vladimin Pshkin, V.A. Medical Center, 921 NE 13th Street, Oklahoma City, Oklahoma 73104
Subscription Rate: $50 Institution, $25 Individual
Circulation/Frequency: 2,500/Quarterly
Pages per Issue: 225
Author Payment: None
Photo Policy: Photos Not Accepted
Writer's Guidelines: American Psychological Association Style Manual
Scope of Journal: Recent research in clinical psychology.

Journal of Community Health
Year of Origin: 1974
Publisher: Human Science Press, 72 Fifth Avenue, New York, New York 10011. Tel: 212 243 6000
Editor: Nemat Borhani, M.D.
Subscription Rate: $78 Institution, $32 Individual
Circulation/Frequency: 1,975/Quarterly
Pages per Issue: 96 average
Author Payment: None
Photo Policy: Black and White Glossies

Writer's Guidelines: No Specific Guidelines; Use Format Within Journal
Scope of Journal: This journal devotes itself to original articles on the practice, teaching, and research of community health and encompasses the areas of preventive medicine, new forms of health manpower, analysis of environmental factors, delivery of health care services, and the study of health maintenance and health insurance programs. Serving as a forum for the exchange of ideas and clarification, the journal features articles on projects which are making an impact on education of health personnel.

Journal of Community Psychology
Year of Origin: 1973
Publisher: Clinical Psychology Publishing Co., Inc., 4 Conant Square, Brandon, Vermont 05733. Tel: 802 247 6871
Editor: J. R. Newbrough, Box 40, Peabody College, Nashville, Tennessee 37203
Subscription Rate: $65 Institution, $25 Individual
Circulation/Frequency: 1,000/Quarterly
Pages per Issue: 100
Author Payment: None
Photo Policy: Photos Not Accepted
Writer's Guidelines: American Psychological Association Style Manual
Scope of Journal: Recent research in community psychology.

Journal of Consulting and Clinical Psychology
Year of Origin: 1968
Publisher: American Psychological Association, 1200 17th Street, NW, Washington, D. C. 20036. Tel: 202 833 7686
Editor: Sol. L. Garfield

Subscription Rate: $25 one-year member, $50 one-year nonmember
Circulation/Frequency: 10,360/Bimonthly
Pages per Issue: 6–7
Author Payment: None
Photo Policy: Black and White Glossies
Scope of Journal: Publishes original contributions and case studies on the development, validity, and use of techniques of diagnosis and treatment in disordered behavior; studies of populations of clinical interest including hospitals, prisons, rehabilitation centers, etc.; cross-cultural studies of behavior disorders; and studies of personality and its assessment and development with regard to problems of consulting and clinical psychology.

The Journal of Continuing Education in Nursing
Year of Origin: 1970
Publisher: Charles B. Slack, Inc., 6900 Grove Road, Thorofare, New Jersey 08086. Tel: 609 848 1000
Editor: Donna Carpenter
Subscription Rate: $22 one-year
Circulation/Frequency: 4,000/Bi-monthly
Pages per Issue: 52
Author Payment: None
Photo Policy: Photos Not Accepted
Scope of Journal: The purposes of this journal are: to bring together a body of literature pertinent to inservice and continuing education needs of nurses; to inform readers of trends in education and health care; to report program designs and educational approaches; to explore issues and problems in inservice and continuing education in nursing; to provide self-learning study units; to seek out and report significant research findings regarding continuing education in nursing.

Journal of Counseling Psychology
Year of Origin: 1954
Publisher: American Psychological Association, 1200 17th Avenue, NW, Washington, D. C. 20036. Tel: 202 833 7686
Editor: Charles J. Gelso
Subscription Rate: $14 one year member, $30 one year nonmember
Circulation/Frequency: 6,000/Bimonthly
Pages per Issue: 7–8
Author Payment: None
Photo Policy: Black and White Glossies
Scope of Journal: Publishes articles on counseling of interest to psychologists and counselors in schools, colleges, universities, private and public counseling agencies, and business, religious, and military settings.

Journal of Divorce
Year of Origin: 1977
Publisher: Haworth Publishing Company, 28 East 22nd Street, New York, New York 10010. Tel: 212 228 2800
Editor: Craig A. Everett, Director, Conciliation Court, Marital and Family Therapy, 111 West Congress, 2nd Floor, Tucson, Arizona 85701
Subscription Date: $28 one-year Individual, $48 one-year Institution, $65 one-year Library
Circulation/Frequency: 1,250/Quarterly
Pages per Issue: Variable
Author Payment: None
Photo Policy: Photos Not Accepted
Writer's Guidelines: Contact Editor
Scope of Journal: A valuable and practical resource for marriage and family counselors and other health professionals. Considers articles dealing with developments in this specific field of interest.

Journal of Drug Education

Year of Origin: 1970
Publisher: Baywood Publishing Company, 120 Marine Street, Box D, Farmingdale, New York 11735. Tel: 516 249 2464
Editor: Seymour Eiseman, Dr. PH, California State University, Northridge, California 91330.
Subscription Rate: $51 Institution, $25 Individual
Circulation/Frequency: 500/Quarterly
Pages per Issue: about 96
Author Payment: None
Photo Policy: Black and White Glossies
Scope of Journal: Pertinent peer-refereed sources of information and ideas for school administrators, supervisors, counselors, teachers, psychologists, health professionals, Armed Forces education and medical officers. Relevant data addressed to the broad spectrum of issues and trends leading to more effective drug education payments.

Journal of Drug Issues

Year of Origin: 1970
Publisher: School of Criminology, Florida State University, Box 4021, Tallahassee, Florida 32303. Tel: 904 385 6524
Editor: Richard L. Rachin
Subscription Rate: $35/year
Circulation/Frequency: 2,500/Quarterly
Pages per Issue: About 130
Author Payment: None
Photo Policy: Photos Not Accepted
Writer's Guidelines: Contact Editor
Scope of Journal: An authoritative review of the social, legal, medical and economic ramifications of drug policy issues.

The Journal of Educational Research

Year of Origin: 1920
Publisher: Heldref Publications, 4000 Albemarle Street NW, Washington, D. C. 20016. Tel: 202 362 6445
Editor: Frank C. Turley
Subscription Rate: $22 one-year
Circulation/Frequency: 3,800/Bimonthly
Pages per Issue: about 64
Author Payment: None
Photo Policy: Camera Ready Accepted
Scope of Journal: This journal publishes manuscripts that describe or synthesize research of direct relevance to educational practice, particularly in elementary and secondary schools. Special consideration is given to articles that focus on variables that can be manipulated in educational settings. Rigorous assessments of the validities of claims for products, testing materials, and educational practices are of particular interest.

Journal of Educational Statistics

Year of Origin: 1976
Publisher: American Educational Research Association, 1230 17th Street NW, Washington, D. C. 20036. Tel: 202 223 9485
Editor: Kris Gilder, 1230 17th Street NW, Washington, D. C. 20036. Tel: 202 223 9485
Subscription Rate: $20 Institution (2 yrs $36), $15 Individual (2 yrs $27)
Circulation/Frequency: 14,000/Quarterly
Pages per Issue: 60–80
Author Payment: None
Photo Policy: Photos Not Accepted
Writer's Guidelines: Upon Request From AERA
Scope of Journal: Demonstrates, primarily through concrete example, how the educational statistician can

contribute to sound, productive, and creative educational decision making and practice. The broad range of disciplines represented are: education, sociology, psychology, history, political science, anthropology, law, economics, philosophy, and statistics.

Journal of Emergency Nursing
Year of Origin: 1975
Publisher: The C. V. Mosby Company, 11830 Westline Industrial Drive, St. Louis, Missouri 63141. Tel: 314 872-8370
Editor: Gail Plsarcik, RN, MS, CS, 666 North Lake Shore Drive, Chicago, Illinois 60611. Tel: 312 649 0297
Subscription Rate: $37.50 one-year Institution USA, $42 International, $16.50 one-year Individual USA, $21 International, $13.20 one-year Student USA, $17.70 International
Circulation/Frequency: 16,344/Bi-monthly
Pages per Issue: 58
Author Payment: None
Photo Policy: Black and White Glossies
Scope of Journal: The official journal of Emergency Department Nurses Association. Articles submitted for publication should represent original communications related to this title and submitted exclusively to this journal.

Journal of Enterostomal Therapy
Year of Origin: 1973
Publisher: The C. V. Mosby Company, 11830 Westline Industrial Drive, St. Louis, Missouri 63141. Tel: 314 872 8370
Editor: Victor Alterescu, RN, ET
Subscription Rate: $43.50 one-year Institution USA, $48.75 International, $22.50 one-year Individual USA, $27.75 International, $18 one-year Student USA, $23.25 International
Circulation/Frequency: 2,000/Bi-monthly
Pages per Issue: 50
Author Payment: None
Photo Policy: Black and White Glossies
Scope of Journal: This journal is a refereed publication designed to meet the continuing educational needs of the International Association for Enterostomal Therapy and the worldwide community of enterostomal therapists. Articles submitted should be original communications related to the title and submitted exclusively to this journal.

Journal of Environmental Health
Year of Origin: 1939
Publisher: National Environmental Health Assoc., 1200 Lincoln Street, Suite 704, Denver, Colorado 80203. Tel: 303 861 9090
Editor: Ida F. Marshall
Subscription Rate: $25 one year (with membership)
Circulation/Frequency: 6,083/Bimonthly
Pages per Issue: 48–56
Author Payment: None
Photo Policy: Black and White Glossies
Scope of Journal: Articles published in all areas of pollution control: health protection in air, land, water, food, waste, water supply and disposal, community sanitation and safety, etc. Reviewed by peers before acceptance. Regular features include an International Viewpoint column, Law for Environmentalists, Audio Visual Reviews; includes news items from governmental agencies, organizations, and industries.

Journal of Family Law
Year of Origin: 1962
Publisher: The University of Louis-
ville, School of Law, Belnap Campus,
Louisville, Kentucky 40292. Tel: 502
588 6396
Editor: Pat Welsh
Subscription Rate: $15 one year
Circulation/Frequency: 1,110/Quar-
terly
Pages per Issue: 200
Author Payment: None
Photo Policy: Photos Not Accepted
Scope of Journal: Articles on all aspects of family law examining current
and emerging issues as well as articles
dealing with historical and theoretical
aspects of domestic relations. Articles
are welcome dealing with family law
related medical-legal subjects, e.g.
paternity testing, abortion legislation,
child abuse, sterilization, etc.

The Journal of Family Welfare
Year of Origin: 1950
Publisher: Family Planning Associa-
tion of India, Bajaj Bhavan, Nariman
Plant, Bombay—400021
Editor: Avabai B. Wadia
Subscription Rate: $5 one-year, £2
one-year
Circulation/Frequency: 4,500/Quar-
terly
Pages per Issue: 85–95
Author Payment: None
Photo Policy: 3 × 4 Black and White
Glossies
Writer's Guidelines: Contact Editor
Scope of Journal: Publishes a variety
of articles on all aspects of family
planning including social, cultural
and demographic factors, maternal
and child health, methods of fertility
control and education for marriage
and family living.

Journal of Food Technology
Publisher: Blackwell Scientific Publica-
tions Ltd., Osney Mead, Oxford OX
2 OEL, England. Tel: 0865 40201
Editor: H. Liebmann, 1FST, 105-111
Euston Street, London NW 1 2ED,
England
Subscription Rate: $195 one-year
USA & Canada
Circulation/Frequency: 2,910/6 yearly
Pages per Issue: about 110
Author Payment: None
Photo Policy: Black and White Glos-
sies Accepted
Writer's Guidelines: Contact Editor
Scope of Journal: The scope of arti-
cles published in this journal range
from pure research in the various sci-
ences associated with food to practical
experiments designed to improve tech-
nical processes.

**Journal of Gerontological Social
Work**
Year of Origin: 1978
Publisher: Haworth Publishing Com-
pany, 28 East 22nd Street, New
York, New York 10010. Tel: 212 228
2800
Editor: Rose Dobrof, Director, Brook-
dale Center on Aging, Hunter Col-
lege, 129 East 79 Street, New York,
New York 10021
Subscription Rate: $28 one-year Indi-
vidual, $48 one-year Institution, $65
one-year Library
Circulation/Frequency: 3,200/Quar-
terly
Pages per Issue: Variable
Author Payment: None
Photo Policy: Photos Not Accepted
Writer's Guidelines: Contact Editor
Scope of Journal: Designed to speak
to social workers and other health
professionals who serve older people;
it does so with the quiet and judi-
cious tone of careful research and

balanced scrutiny. Quality is ensured through selection procedures of an Editorial Board.

The Journal of Hand Surgery
Year of Origin: 1976
Publisher: C. V. Mosby Company, 11830 Westline Industrial Drive, St. Louis, Missouri 63141. Tel: 314 872 8370
Editor: Adrian E. Flatt, MD, Department of Surgery, Norwalk Hospital, Norwalk, Connecticut 06856. Tel: 203 852 2390
Subscription Rate: $47 one-year Institution USA, $52.75 International, $26 one-year Individual USA, $31.75 International, $20.80 one-year Student USA, $26.55 International
Circulation/Frequency: 7,431/Bimonthly
Pages per Issue: 115
Author Payment: None
Photo Policy: Black and White Glossies 5 × 7
Scope of Journal: This journal is directed to the surgeon who seeks to restore function of the hand and upper extremity regardless of the cause of the impairment. From an operative standpoint, the hand surgeon is a combination of orthopedic, plastic, vascular and neurosurgeon. This journal is the official publication of The American Society for Surgery of the Hand.

Journal of Health Politics, Policy and Law
Year of Origin: 1976
Publisher: Department of Health Administration, Duke University, Box 3018, Duke Medical Center, Durham, North Carolina 27710. Tel: 919 984 4188
Editor: T. R. Marmor, 15A Yale Station, New Haven, Connecticut 06520
Subscription Rate: $48 Institution,

$32 Individual, $16 Student
Circulation/Frequency: 1,600/Quarterly
Pages per Issue: 260
Author Payment: None
Photo Policy: Photos Not Accepted
Scope of Journal: This journal publishes the work of scholars, policymakers, and practitioners whose interests bear broadly on health. Lively, concise articles from any disciplinary perspective and from anywhere in the world are welcome.

Journal of Holistic Medicine
Year of Origin: 1978
Publisher: Human Sciences Press, Inc., 72 Fifth Avenue, New York, New York 10011. Tel: 212 243 6783
Editor: Elmer Cranton, M.D.
Subscription Rate: $18 one-year Individual, $40 one-year Institution
Circulation/Frequency: 2,000/4 yearly
Pages per Issue: 96
Author Payment: None
Photo Policy: Black and white Glossies
Writer's Guidelines: No Specific Guidelines; Use Format Within Journal
Scope of Journal: The contributors illustrate that holistic medicine encompasses all safe modalities of diagnosis and treatment, including drugs and surgery, emphasizing the necessity of looking at the whole person through an analysis of physical, nutritional, environmental, emotional, spiritual, and life style values.

The Journal of Homosexuality
Year of Origin: 1981
Publisher: The Haworth Press, Inc., 28 East 22nd Street, New York, New York 10010. Tel: 212 228 2800
Editor: John P. DeCecco, C.E.R.E.S., Psychology Bldg., Room 503, San Franscisco State University, San Fran-

cisco, California 94132. Tel: 415 569 1137
Subscription Rate: $32 USA/Canada/ Mexico Individual, $60 USA/Canada/ Mexico Institution, $80 USA/Canada/Mexico Library, $42 Foreign Individual, $80 Foreign Institution, $110 Foreign Library
Circulation/Frequency: Unavailable/Quarterly
Pages per Issue: Variable
Author Payment: None
Photo Policy: Photos Not Accepted
Writer's Guidelines: Contact Editor
Scope of Journal: Devoted entirely to the study of homosexuality, theme-oriented issues.

Journal of Housing For The Elderly
Year of Origin: 1983
Publisher: Haworth Publishing Company, 28 East 22nd Street, New York, New York 10010. Tel: 212 228 2800
Editor: Leon Pastelan, Co-Director, National Policy Center on Housing and Living Arrangements for Older Americans, University of Michigan, 2000 Bonisteel Blvd., Lansing, Michigan 48924
Subscription Rate: $34 one-year Individual, $48 one-year Institution, $65 one-year Library
Circulation/Frequency: Unavailable/Quarterly
Pages per Issue: Variable
Author Payment: None
Photo Policy: Photos Not Accepted
Writer's Guidelines: Contact Editor
Scope of Journal: The goal of this journal is the rapid publication of new research in the housing and aging fields, plus the synthesizing of the cross-disciplinary efforts being made to enhance the residential environments of the elderly.

Journal of Hygiene
Year of Origin: 1901
Publisher: Cambridge University Press, 32 East 57th Street, New York, New York 10022. Tel: 212 688 8885
Editor: Prof. J. R. Pattison, Prof. W. C. Noble, Dr. Malcolm Lewis, Dr. J. H. Mc Coy
Subscription Rate: $160 one-year
Circulation/Frequency: 1,429 yearly/ Bimonthly
Pages per Issue: 175
Author Payment: None
Photo Policy: Black and White Glossies
Scope of Journal: This journal publishes reports and research in subjects related to hygiene and preventive and social medicine. It is concerned with the control of infectious disease in the community.

Journal of Immunogenetics
Publisher: Blackwell Scientific Publications, Ltd., Osney Mead, Oxford, OX 2 OLL
Editor: Dr. K. Bauer, Privatdozent, Postfach 10 15 60, D-6900, Heidelberg 1, West Germany
Subscription Rate: £52 one-year UK, £62.50 one-year Overseas, $145 one-year USA
Circulation/Frequency: 630/Bi-monthly
Pages per Issue: about 25
Author Payment: None
Photo Policy: Black and White Glossies
Writer's Guidelines: Contact Editor
Scope of Journal: Designed to provide a common forum for scientists working in the various fields that contribute to the understanding of immunogenetics. Its scope includes the immunogenetics of antigens in man, of antibodies, the immune response and the complement system.

Journal of Infectious Diseases
Year of Origin: 1968
Publisher: University of Chicago
Press, Room 151, University of Illinois Hospitals, 1853 West Polk
Street, Chicago, Illinois 60612. Tel.
312 996 7890
Editor: George Jackson, MD
Subscription Rate: $115 Institution,
$57 Individual, $30 Student
Circulation/Frequency: 8,000/Monthly
Pages per Issue: 160
Author Payment: None
Photo Policy: Glossy Prints not to exceed 8½ × 11
Scope of Journal: Reports of research
and reviews related to any aspect of
the fields of microbiology and infection whether laboratory, clinical or
epidemiologic are welcome. Focus is
on pathogenesis, clinical investigation,
medical microbiology, diagnosis and/
or treatment of diseases caused by infectious agents or abnormal
conditions in the host, and immune
mechanisms.

Journal of International Medical Research
Publisher: Cambridge Medical Publications Ltd, 435/437 Wellingborough
Rd, Northampton NN1 4EZ, England
Editor: Dr. Eric Murphy
Subscription Rate: $60 one-year
Circulation/Frequency: 6,000/6 yearly
Pages per Issue: 60-120
Author Payment: 65% contributed
Photo Policy: 3 × 5 Black and White
Glossies
Scope of Journal: Publishes the results of pharmaceutical research and
original papers of clinical importance.

The Journal of Laboratory and Clinical Medicine
Year of Origin: 1915
Publisher: The C. V. Mosby Company, 11830 Westline Industrial

Drive, St. Louis, Missouri 63141. Tel:
314 872 8370
Editor: Charles E. Mengel, MD, Department of Medicine, N-424, University of Missouri Health Sciences,
Columbia, Missouri 65212. Tel: 314
882 1513
Subscription Rate: $62 one-year Institution USA, $74 International, $41
one-year Individual USA, $53 International, $32.80 one-year Student
USA, $44.80 International
Circulation/Frequency: 5,638/Monthly
Pages per Issue: 160
Author Payment: None
Photo Policy: Black and White Glossies 5 × 7 or less
Scope of Journal: This journal is directed to directors of clinical and
pathology laboratories, laboratory
consultants, laboratory technologists
interested in advanced information,
physicians especially interested in
diagnosis, and those with a related
interest in investigation and research.

Journal of Learning Disabilities
Year of Origin: 1968
Publisher: William N. Topaz, Professional Press, Inc., 101 East Ontario
Street, Chicago, Illinois 60611
Editor: Gerald M. Senf, Ph.D., 1331
East Thunderhead Drive, Tucson,
Arizona 85718. Tel: 602 297 2842
Subscription Rate: $27 one-year USA,
$34 one-year Canada, $40 one-year
Foreign
Circulation/Frequency: 15,000/ten
yearly
Pages per Issue: 72
Author Payment: free
Photo Policy: Camera Ready Accepted
Writer's Guidelines: Contact Editor
Scope of Journal: This journal is a
multidisciplinary publication containing articles on practice, research, and
theory related to learning disabilities.

It includes reports of research, opinion papers, case reports, and discussion of issues which are the concern of all disciplines engaged in the field. Book reviews and letters to the editor are welcome.

Journal of Marital and Family Therapy

Year of Origin: 1975
Publisher: American Association for Marriage and Family Therapy, 924 West 9th Street, Upland, California 91786
Editor: Alan S. Gurman, Ph.D.
Subscription Rate: $20 one-year Individual, $30 one-year Institution
Circulation/Frequency: 12,000/Quarterly
Pages per Issue: 100
Author Payment: None
Photo Policy: Photos Not Accepted
Scope of Journal: This journal offers broad coverage of recent news developments in the field of marriage and family therapy, and is published to advance the professional understanding of marital and family behavior. Also, the journal aims to improve the psychotherapeutic treatment of marital and family dysfunction.

Journal of Marriage and the Family

Year of Origin: 1939
Publisher: National Council on Family Relations
Editor: Jetse Sprety, Ph.D., Department of Sociology, Case Western Reserve University, Cleveland, Ohio 44106. Tel: 216 368 2705
Subscription Rate: $30 one-year Individual, $35 one-year Institution, $50 one-year NCFR Membership journal included
Circulation/Frequency: 9,000/Quarterly
Pages per Issue: 220
Author Payment: None

Photo Policy: 6 × 9 Black and White Glossies
Writer's Guidelines: Contact Editor
Scope of Journal: This journal is a vehicle for theory and research in the area of marriage and the family; its focus is interdisciplinary.

The Journal of Medicine and Philosophy

Year of Origin: 1976
Publisher: The Catholic University of America, Washington D. C. 20064, USA
Editor: D. Reidel, Box 17, 3300 AA Dordrecht, Holland
Subscription Rate: $33 USA Institution, $18 USA Individual
Circulation/Frequency: 2,400/Quarterly
Pages per Issue: 96
Author Payment: None
Photo Policy: Photos Not Accepted
Scope of Journal: This publication has been established under the auspices of the Society for Health and Human Values to explore the shared themes and concerns of philosophy and the medical sciences. Central issues in medical research and practice have important philosophical dimensions, for in treating disease and promoting health, medicine involves presuppositions about human goals and values. Conversely, the concerns of philosophy often significantly relate to those of medicine.

Journal of Mental Deficiency Research

Year of Origin: 1957
Publisher: Blackwell Scientific Publications Ltd, 8 John Street, London, WC1N 2ES, England
Editor: B. W. Richards, St. Lawrence's Hospital, Caterham, Surrey, England
Subscription Rate: $62.50 one-year

USA & Canada
Circulation/Frequency: 1,100/Quarterly
Pages per Issue: about 80
Author Payment: None
Photo Policy: Black and White Glossies Accepted
Writer's Guidelines: Contact Editor
Scope of Journal: Publishes articles on medical and psychological research with occasional reviews of current progress. The scope includes clinical case reports and prevalence studies, pathology, and any topic which may be of relevance to the diagnosis, prevention and treatment of mental subnormality.

The Journal of Neuro-Oncology
Year of Origin: 1982
Publisher: Martinus Nijhoff, Box 566, 2501 CN The Hague, The Netherlands. Tel: 070 469 460
Editor: Michael D. Walker, MD
Subscription Rate: $48 one-year Individual USA, $80 one-year Institution USA, (Airmail add $9)
Circulation/Frequency: New/Quarterly
Pages per Issue: 80–100
Author Payment: None
Photo Policy: Photos Not Accepted
Scope of Journal: A multi-disciplinary journal encompassing basic, applied and clinical investigation in all research areas as they relate to cancer and the central nervous system. This journal does not seek to isolate the field, but rather to focus the efforts of many disciplines in one publication.

Journal of Neurophysiology
Year of Origin: 1938
Publisher: American Physiological Society, 9650 Rockville Pike, Bethesda, Maryland 20014. Tel: 301 530 7160
Editor: Stephen R. Geiger
Subscription Rate: $110 USA, $130

Foreign
Circulation/Frequency: Unavailable/Monthly
Pages per Issue: about 400
Author Payment: None
Photo Policy: Black and White Glossies
Scope of Journal: Publishes original articles on the function of the nervous system. Approaches used to elucidate nervous system function can include electrophysiology, experimental neuroanatomy and electron microscopy, neurochemistry, cellular neurobiology, developmental neurobiology, tissue culture, and behavioral analysis.

Journal of Nonverbal Behavior
Year of Origin: 1976
Publisher: Human Science Press, 72 Fifth Avenue, New York, New York 10011. Tel: 212 243 6000
Editor: Randolph M. Lee
Subscription Rate: $58 Institution, $26 Individual
Circulation/Frequency: 1,050/Quarterly
Pages per Issue: 64 average
Author Payment: None
Photo Policy: Black and White Glossies
Writer's Guidelines: No Specific Guidelines; use Format Within Journal
Scope of Journal: This journal presents original theoretical and empirical research on all major areas of nonverbal behavior. Specific areas include paralanguage, proxemics, facial expressions, eye contact, face-to-face interaction, nonverbal emotional expression, as well as other areas which increase the scientific understanding of nonverbal processes and behavior. Studies from related fields including anthropology, sociology, and linguistics are considered.

The Journal of Nursing Administration
Year of Origin: 1970
Publisher: Concept Development,
Inc., 12 Lakeside Park, Wakefield,
Massachusetts 10880. Tel: 617 246
3130; 617 245 4736
Editor: Carol Higgins Rougvie
Subscription Rate: $24.95 one-year
Circulation/Frequency:
14,000/Monthly
Pages per issue: 50
Author payment: None; 2 com-
plimentary copies
Photo Policy: Photos Not Accepted
Scope of Journal: JONA is a manage-
ment journal edited and published
specifically for chief nursing execu-
tives. Articles range from the theoret-
ical to the "how-to-do-it." JONA also
contains special features that offer
material from a variety of sources for
health professionals.

The Journal of Nursing Care
Year of Origin: 1967
Publisher: Mel Kohudic, 265 Post
Road West, Box 913, Westport, Con-
necticut 06881. Tel: 203 226 7203
Editor: Jerry C. Melson
Subscription Rate: $12 one-year
Circulation/Frequency:
12,000/Monthly
Pages per Issue: about 24
Author Payment: 80% contributed
Photo Policy: Black and White Glos-
sies, 8 × 10
Scope of Journal: This is the largest
independent journal for the licensed
practical nurse and covers clinical as-
pects, articles of special interest to
the bedside nurse, geriatric care,
pediatric care and profiles of the
LPN's.

Journal of Nursing Education
Year of Origin: 1961
Publisher: Charles B. Slack, Inc.,
6900 Grove Road, Thorofare, New
Jersey, 08086. Tel: 609 848 1000
Editor: Margaret Carnine, RN
Subscription Rate: $20 one-year
Circulation/Frequency: 3,461/9 each
year
Pages per Issue: 48
Author Payment: None
Photo Policy: Photos Not Accepted
Scope of Journal: This journal ac-
cepts original articles of interest to
nurses working in the field of educa-
tion.

Journal of Nutrition
Year of Origin: 1928
Publisher: The American Institution
of Nutrition, 9650 Rockville Pike,
Bethesda, Maryland 20814
Editor: Dr. James S. Dinning, 427
Food Science Bldg., University of
Florida, Gainesville, Florida 32611.
Tel: 904 392 2559
Subscription Rate: $60 one-year Indi-
vidual, $72 one-year Institution
Circulation/Frequency: 4,500/Monthly
Pages per Issue: about 200
Author Payment: None
Photo Policy: Photos Not Accepted
Scope of Journal: This journal con-
tains concise reports of original re-
search bearing on the nature of food
nutrients and the function in a va-
riety of organisms, and articles which
report the development of new nutritional concepts and interrelationships
of importance in human and animal
nutrition.

Journal of Nutrition Education
Year of Origin: 1968
Publisher: Helen Ullrich, 1736 Frank-
lin Street, Ninth Floor, Oakland, Cali-
fornia 94612. Tel: 415 444 7133
Editor: Susan M. Oace

Subscription Rate: $25 Individual USA, $27 Individual Foreign, $30 Institution USA, $32 Institution Foreign, $8, Single Copy USA, $8.50 Single Copy Foreign
Circulation/Frequency: 8,000/Quarterly
Pages per Issue: 48
Author Payment: None
Photo Policy: Photos Not Accepted
Scope of Journal: This Journal is refereed and designed to stimulate interest and research in applied nutritional sciences and to disseminate information to educators and others concerned about positive nutritional practices and policies. Concise reports of original research and reviews relevant to nutrition education, short articles presenting viewpoints on current issues and controversies in nutrition education or reporting creative program ideas are welcome.

Journal of Nutrition for the Elderly
Year of Origin: 1980
Publisher: Haworth Publishing Company, 28 East 22nd Street, New York, New York 10010. Tel: 212 228 2800
Editor: Annette B. Natow, School of Nursing, Adelphi University, Garden City, New York 11530
Subscription Rate: $28 one-year Individual, $48 one-year Institution, $65 one-year Library
Circulation/Frequency: 1,350/Quarterly
Pages per Issue: Variable
Author Payment: None
Photo Policy: Photos Not Accepted
Writer's Guidelines: Contact Editor
Scope of Journal: This journal is devoted to nutritional services, research, programs, and care for the elderly; it is directed to dieticians, nutritionists and other health professionals concerned with long-term care.

Journal of Obesity and Weight Regulation
Year of Origin: 1980
Publisher: Human Sciences Press, Inc., 72 Fifth Avenue, New York, New York 10011. Tel: 212 243 6783
Editor: Jonathan Wise, M. D., Robert Sherwin, M. D.
Subscription Rate: $30 one-year Individual, $76 one-year Institution
Circulation/Frequency: 500/ 4 yearly
Pages per Issue: 64
Author Payment: None
Photo Policy: Black and White Glossies
Writer's Guidelines: No Specific Guidelines; Use Format Within Journal
Scope of Journal: This journal presents an interdisciplinary forum solely devoted to the scientific study of obesity. Obesity can be fully understood and treated only when it is viewed in its medical, psychological, and social context. Articles in this journal examine all major clinical as well as theoretical approaches to problems in obesity.

Journal of Obstetric, Gynecologic and Neonatal Nursing
Year of Origin: 1969
Publisher: Lippincott/Harper, East Washington Square, Philadelphia, Pennsylvania 19105. Tel: 215 574 4200
Editor: Judith Serevino, 600 Maryland Avenue SW, Suite 200, Washington, D. C. 20024
Subscription Rate: $20 one-year
Circulation/Frequency: 24,000/Bimonthly
Pages per Issue: 64
Author Payment: None
Photo Policy: Black and White Glossies, 8 × 10
Scope of Journal: This is the official journal of the Nurses Association of

The American College of Obstetricians and Gynecologists and is designed to reflect thought, trends, policies, and research in obstetric, gynecologic, and neonatal nursing. Research papers and other articles which incorporate views, experience, and knowledge in these areas will be considered.

Journal of Operational Psychiatry
Year of Origin: 1970
Publisher: University of Missouri—Columbia, Department of Psychiatry, 803 Stadium Road, Columbia, Missouri 65201. Tel: 314 445 1242
Editor: Armando Favazza, M. D.
Subscription Rate: $10 one year, (Free to Psychiatrists)
Circulation/Frequency: 28,000/Monthly
Pages per Issue: 100
Author Payment: None
Photo Policy: Photos Not Accepted
Writer's Guidelines: Contact Publisher
Scope of Journal: Publishes articles of interest to psychiatrists and other health professionals. Highest priority is given to articles of an interdisciplinary nature, e. g. psychiatry/anthropology/sociology/psychology.

Journal of Occupational Medicine
Year of Origin: 1959
Publisher: Doris L. Flournoy, 1845 West Morse, Chicago, Illinois 60626. Tel: 312 761 3955
Editor: Lloyd B. Tepper, MD
Subscription Rate: $25 one-year
Circulation/Frequency: 7,700/Monthly
Pages per Issue: 72–104
Author Payment: None
Photo Policy: Black and White Glossies
Scope of Journal: This journal publishes original articles on such topics as industrial toxicology, occupational medical practice, epidemiology of occupational disease, ergonomics, radiation health, surgery of trauma, occupational health administration, assessment of disability, rehabilitation, mental health in injury, audiology, health education, pulmonary function and occupational lung disease, health screening, occupational dermatology and health data management.

Journal of Ophthalmic Nursing and Technology
Year of Origin: 1982
Publisher: Charles B. Slack, Inc., 6900 Grove Road, Thorofare, New Jersey, 08086. Tel: 609 848 1000
Editor: Patricia L. Zack, RN
Subscription Rate: $15 one-year
Circulation/Frequency: 780/Quarterly
Pages per Issue: 48
Author Payment: None
Photo Policy: Black and White Glossies Accepted
Scope of Journal: This journal includes articles of interest to registered nurses specializing in ophthalmology and technologists in the field of ophthalmology.

Journal of Oral and Maxillofacial Surgery
Previously: **Journal of Oral Surgery**
Year of Origin: 1943
Publisher: W. B. Saunders Company, West Washington Square, Philadelphia, Pennsylvania 19105. Tel: 215 574 4859
Editor: Daniel M. Laskin, D.D.S.
Subscription Rate: $42 one-year Institution, $35 one-year Individual (Add $7 foreign delivery; $25 air mail)
Circulation/Frequency: 8,500/Monthly
Pages per Issue: 64
Author Payment: None
Photo Policy: Photos Not Accepted
Scope of Journal: This journal serves oral and maxillofacial surgeons, gen-

eral practitioners, schools, hospitals, and dental departments with a special interest in oral surgery. The journal publishes scientific articles, case reports, editorials and news in the field of oral surgery.

Journal of Organizational Behavior Management
Year of Origin: 1977
Publisher: Haworth Publishing Company, 28 East 22nd Street, New York, New York 10010. Tel: 212 228 2800
Editor: Lee W. Frederiksen, Director, Psychological Services Center, Department of Psychology, Virginia Polytechnic Institute, Blacksburg, Virginia 24061
Subscription Rate: $32 one-year Individual, $48 one-year Institution, $65 one-year Library
Circulation/Frequency: 1,400/Quarterly
Pages per Issue: Variable
Author Payment: None
Photo Policy: Photos Not Accepted
Writer's Guidelines: Contact Editor
Scope of Journal: Behavior management principles in the industrial and organizational setting; data-based research dealing with applied behavior analysis . . . the practical aspects of program design, implementation, and continued assessment.

Journal of Pediatric Ophthalmology and Strabismus
Year of Origin: 1963
Publisher: Charles B. Slack, Inc., 6900 Grove Road, Thorofare, New Jersey 08086. Tel: 609 848 1000
Editor: Henry S. Metz, MD
Subscription Rate: $36 one-year
Circulation/Frequency: 1,332/Bi-monthly
Pages per Issue: 56
Author Payment: None

Photo Policy: Black and White Glossies
Scope of Journal: This journal publishes articles of interest to physicians specializing in the practice of pediatric ophthalmology and/or strabismus and pediatrics.

The Journal of Pediatrics
Year of Origin: 1932
Publisher: The C. V. Mosby Company, 11830 Westline Industrial Drive, St. Louis, Missouri 63141. Tel: 314 872 8370
Editor: Joseph M. Garfunkel, MD, Box 3307, Springfield, Illinois 62708. Tel: 217 789 4204
Subscription Rate: $54.50 one-year Institution USA, $69.75 International, $33.50 one-year Individual USA, $48.75 International, $26.80 one-year Student USA, $42.05 International
Circulation/Frequency: 31.072/Monthly
Pages per Issue: 190
Author Payment: None
Photo Policy: Black and White Glossies
Scope of Journal: The articles submitted for publication should represent original communication relating to this title and be submitted exclusively to The Journal of Pediatrics.

Journal of Personality and Social Psychology
Year of Origin: 1963
Publisher: American Psychological Association, 1200 17th Street, NW, Washington, D. C. 20036. Tel: 202 833 7686
Editor: Melvin Manis: Attitudes & Social Cognition Section, Ivan D. Steiner: Interpersonal Relations and Group Processes Section, Robert Hogan: Personality Processes and Individual Differences Section
Subscription Rate: $35 one-year

member, $90 one-year nonmember
Circulation/Frequency: 6,440/Monthly
Pages per Issue: 11–12
Author Payment: None
Photo Policy: Black and White Glossies
Scope of Journal: Publishes original papers in all areas of personality and social psychology. It emphasizes empirical reports but may include specialized theoretical, methodological, and review papers. The three sections cover papers dealing with the formation or change of beliefs or attitudes, measurement of attitudes, and the relation between attitudes and behavior; the interaction between two or more people; and aspects of personality psychology as traditionally defined.

Journal of Physiology
Year of Origin: 1878
Publisher: Cambridge University Press, 32 East 57th Street, New York, New York 10022. Tel: 212 688 8885
Editor: Professor S. Thomas
Subscription Rate: $880
Circulation/Frequency: 3,532/Monthly
Pages per Issue: 656 per volume
Author Payment: None
Photo Policy: Photos Not Accepted
Scope of Journal: This journal is concerned with all aspects of physiological research: respiration, circulation, excretion, reproduction, digestion, homeostasis, and particularly neurophysiology and muscular contraction. In addition to original articles, it publishes the proceedings of the Physiological Society.

Journal of Prison and Jail Health
Year of Origin: 1980
Publisher: Human Science Press, Inc., 72 Fifth Avenue, New York, New York 10011. Tel: 212 243 6783
Editor: Nancy Neveloff Dubler, L.L.B.

Subscription Rate: $19 one-year Individual, $40 one-year Institution
Circulation/Frequency: 400/4 yearly
Pages per Issue: 64
Author Payment: None
Photo Policy: Black and White Glossies
Writer's Guidelines: No Specific Guidelines; Use Format Within Journal
Scope of Journal: This journal is addressed to physicians, prison health professionals, lawyers, inmate advocates, and correctional managers; this journal marks the first publication solely devoted to discussions of health maintenance and self-care among inmates.

The Journal of Prosthetic Dentistry
Year of Origin: 1951
Publisher: The C. V. Mosby Company, 11830 Westline Industrial Drive, St. Louis, Missouri 83141. Tel: 314 872 8370
Editor: Judson C. Hickey, Medical College of Georgia, School of Dentistry, Augusta, Georgia 30912
Subscription Rate: $50.50 one-year Institution USA, $62.50 International, $29.50 one-year Individual USA, $41.50 International, $13.50 one-year Student USA, $25.50 International
Circulation/Frequency: 20,878/Monthly
Pages per Issue: 126
Author Payment: None
Photo Policy: Black and White Glossies
Scope of Journal: This journal represents 20 organizational affiliations associated with prosthetic dentistry. Articles submitted for publication should represent original communication related to this title and be submitted exclusively to this journal.

Journal of Psychiatric Research
Year of Origin: 1961
Publisher: Pergamon Press, Maxwell House, Fairview Park, Elmsford, New York 10523. Tel: 914 592 7700
Editor: Seymour S. Kety, Laboratories for Psychiatric Research, Mailman Research Center, McClear Hospital, Belmont, Massachusetts 02178
Subscription Rate: $120 one-year
Circulation/Frequency: 2,500/Quarterly
Pages per Issue: about 268
Author Payment: None
Photo Policy: Photos Not Accepted
Scope of Journal: This journal was founded as a medium for the communication of the increasing number of research reports of high quality in psychiatry and cognate disciplines. It welcomes original research reports which are well designed and critically controlled relevant to psychiatric problems and representing clinical, biological psychological and sociological areas.

The Journal of Psychology
Year of Origin: 1936
Publisher: The Journal Press, 2 Commercial Street, Box 543, Provincetown, Massachusetts 02657
Editor: Editorial Board
Subscription Rate: $54 one-year
Circulation/Frequency: 1,660/6 yearly
Pages per Issue: 160
Author Payment: None
Photo Policy: Photos Not Accepted
Writer's Guidelines: Contact Publisher
Scope of Journal: This journal includes articles and research which concern general issues in the field of psychology and related fields.

The Journal of Psychosomatic Research
Year of Origin: 1956
Publisher: The Pergamon Press, Maxwell House, Fairview Park, Elmsford, New York 10523. Tel: 914 592 7700
Editor: Cairns Aitken, Rehabilitation Studies Unit, Princess Margaret Rose Hospital, Fairmilehead, Edinburgh, Scotland EH10FED
Subscription Rate: $140 one-year
Circulation/Frequency: 3,000/Bimonthly
Pages per Issue: 80 average
Author Payment: 25 reprints free
Photo Policy: Black and White Glossies
Scope of Journal: Original psychosomatic research not previously published and will not be published elsewhere in any language without consent of the editor.

Journal of Rehabilitation
Publisher: Blackwell Scientific Publications Ltd., Osney Mead, Oxford OX 2 OLL
Editor: A.S.T. Franks, Dental School, University of Birmingham, St. Chads Queensway, Birmingham, B4 6NN
Subscription Rate: $145 one-year USA/Canada, £56 one-year UK
Circulation/Frequency: 500/Bi-monthly
Pages per Issue: 540
Author Payment: None
Photo Policy: Black and White Glossies
Writer's Guidelines: Contact Editor
Scope of Journal: Designed to be of practical use to dental units involved in clinical care, research, and teaching, as well as dental practitioners and other health professionals.

Journal of Religion and Health
Year of Origin: 1960
Publisher: Human Science Press, 72 Fifth Avenue, New York, New York 10011. Tel: 212 243 6000
Editor: Harry C. Meserve
Subscription Rate: $68 Institution, $29 Individual

Circulation/Frequency: 2,000/Quarterly
Pages per Issue: 80 average
Author Payment: None
Photo Policy: Black and White Glossies
Writer's Guidelines: No Specific Guidelines; Use Format Within Journal
Scope of Journal: A journal which critically explores the most contemporary modes of religious thought with particular emphasis on its relevance to current medical and psychological research. This publication provides a scholarly forum for the discussion of topical themes on both a theoretical and a practical level. Issues center on the methods by which the religious viewpoint works cooperatively with specialists in the helping professions with the aim of promoting an ethical and psychologically balanced culture.

Journal of Reproduction and Fertility
Year of Origin: 1960
Publisher: Journals of Reproduction and Fertility Ltd, 22 Newmarket Road, Cambridge, England, CB 5 8 DT. Tel: 0223 51809
Editor: Dr. Barbara J. Weir
Subscription Rate: $210 one-year
Circulation/Frequency: Unavailable/6 yearly
Pages per Issue: 250
Author Payment: None
Photo Policy: Submit unmounted; 2 Monochrome plates free; subsequent plates and color plates charged to author
Scope of Journal: This journal publishes original papers, reviews and bibliographies on the morphology, physiology, biochemistry, and pathology of reproduction in man and other animals, and on the biological and medical problems of fertility and lactation.

Journal of Safety Research
Year of Origin: 1969
Publisher: Pergamon Press, Inc., Maxwell House, Fairview Park, Elmsford, New York 10523. Tel: 914 592 9700
Editor: Thomas W. Planek, Ph.D., Managing Editor: Jean Stephenson, Editorial Asst.: Sharon Crater, Consulting Editors: Joseph Bryk, Alan Hoskin, Kathryn Race
Subscription Rate: $45 one-year; $85 two-year, $28 members
Membership Inquiries: National Safety Council, 444 North Michigan Avenue, Chicago, Illinois 60611. Tel. 312 527 4800, ext. 302
Circulation/Frequency: 4200/Quarterly
Pages per Issue: 40–50
Author Payment: 25 complimentary reprints
Photo Policy: Black and White Glossies
Scope of Journal: This journal is an interdisciplinary publication that provides for the exchange of ideas and data developed through research experience in all areas of safety: traffic, industry, farm, home, school and public. Articles may deal with a variety of topics: human error and accidents, methods of accident investigation and analysis, evaluative examination of accident countermeasures or the relation between man-machine environment factors and hazards.

The Journal of School Health
Year of Origin: 1930
Publisher: American School Health Association, 1521 South Water Street, Kent, Ohio 44240. Tel: 216 678 1601
Editor: Alison Bashian
Subscription Rate: $35 one year

members, $15 one year students/retirees
Circulation/Frequency: 9,000/Monthly
Pages per Issue: 56–64
Author Payment: None
Photo Policy: Camera Ready Copy
Only
Scope of Journal: This journal is a national publication serving school nurses and physicians, health educators, psychologists, dental hygenists and others concerned with school health. Editorial coverage includes administration of health education programs, health problems associated with child development, programs of disease control, sex education, research in child health activities of nurses, dental health, teaching resources, descriptions of actual medican and nursing program, alcohol and drug abuse programs, curriculum construction and preparation of personnel.

Journal of School Psychology
Year of Origin: 1961
Publisher: Human Science Press, 72 Fifth Avenue, New York, New York 10011. Tel: 212 243 6000
Editor: Thomas Oakland
Subscription Rate: $55 Institution, $25 Individual
Circulation/Frequency: 3,300/Quarterly
Pages per Issue: 96 average
Author Payment: None
Photo Policy: Black and White Glossies
Writer's Guidelines: No Specific Guidelines; Use Format Within Journal
Scope of Journal: This journal is intended for psychologists and others working with, or responsible for training programs or psychological services in the schools. This publication includes articles on research,

opinion, and practice with the aim of fostering the continued development of school psychology as an important scientific and professional specialty.

Journal of the Science of Food and Agriculture
Publisher: Blackwell Scientific Publications Ltd, 8 John Street, London WC1N 2ES, England
Editor: E. R. Dinnis, Glebe House, North Cowton, North Yorkshire
Subscription Rate: $125 one-year USA & Canada
Circulation/Frequency: 1,870/Monthly
Pages per Issue: about 120
Author Payment: None
Photo Policy: Black and White Glossies Accepted
Writer's Guidelines: Contact Editor
Scope of Journal: This journal is concerned with: publication of research papers, notes and review articles in the field of food science and other associated sciences. It deals with vegetable, fruit, meat, egg and milk technology together with all branches of agriculture.

The Journal of Sex Research
Year of Origin: 1965
Publisher: The Society for the Scientific Study of Sex
Editor: Clive M. Davis, Ph.D., Department of Psychology, Syracuse University, Syracuse, New York 13210. Tel: 315 423 3658
Subscription Rate: $35 one-year Individual, $50 one-year Institution, $25 one-year Members
Circulation/Frequency: 1,500/Quarterly
Pages per Issue: 96
Author Payment: None
Photo Policy: Camera Ready Copy Accepted
Scope of Journal: This journal serves

as a forum for the interdisciplinary exchange of knowledge among professionals concerned with the scientific study of sexuality. Articles reporting original empirical research, theoretical essays, literature reviews, methodological articles, historical articles, clinical reports, and teaching papers are publishable; book reviews and article reviews will also be considered.

Journal of Social Policy
Year of Origin: 1971
Publisher: Cambridge University Press, 32 East 57th Street, New York, New York 10022. Tel: 212 688 8885
Editor: Ken Judge
Subscription Rate: $52 one-year Individual, $88 one-year Institution
Circulation/Frequency: 1,308 year/Quarterly
Pages per Issue: 176
Author Payment: None
Photo Policy: Photos Not Accepted
Scope of Journal: This journal is an important source of information for scholars and professionals in regard to development and implementation of public programs; income maintenance, health education, housing and urban planning, social services, and social change. It provides a thoughtful critical analysis of controversies and issues of public policy viewed in crossnational terms.

The Journal of Social Psychology
Year of Origin: 1930
Publisher: The Journal Press, 2 Commercial Street, Box 543, Provincetown, Massachusetts 02657. Tel: 617 487 0133
Editor: Leonard W. Doob
Subscription Rate: $54/annual
Circulation/Frequency: 2,375/Bi-monthly
Pages per Issue: 160 average

Author Payment: None
Photo Policy: Photos Not Required
Scope of Journal: This journal is devoted to studies of persons in group settings and of culture and personality; special attention to cross-cultural articles and notes, to field research, and to briefly reported Replications and Refinements.

Journal of Social Work and Human Sexuality
Year of Origin: 1982
Publisher: Haworth Publishing Company, 28 East 22nd Street, New York, New York 10010. Tel: 212 228 2800
Editor: David A. Shore, 2909 North Sheridan Road, Suite 1307, Chicago, Illinois 60657
Subscription Rate: $28 one-year Individual, $36 one-year Institution, $60 one-year Library
Circulation/Frequency: Unavailable/Quarterly
Pages per Issue: Variable
Author Payment: None
Photo Policy: Photos Not Accepted
Writer's Guidelines: Contact Editor
Scope of Journal: This is a new journal directed to sexual issues in social work and for all helping professionals. Articles include material of generic interest to those in the field of human sexuality and involved with the broad range of issues pertaining to sexuality and family planning.

Journal of Speech and Hearing Disorders
Year of Origin: 1936
Publisher: American Speech-Language-Hearing Association, 10801 Rockville Pike, Rockville, Maryland 20853. Tel: 301 897 5700
Subscription Rate: $45 one-year USA, $48 one-year Foreign

Circulation/Frequency: 43,000/Quarterly
Pages per Issue: 112
Author Payment: $65 page charge to author
Photo Policy: Camera Ready Accepted
Writer's Guidelines: American Psychological Association Style Manual
Scope of Journal: This journal pertains to the nature and treatment of disordered speech, hearing, and language and to the clinical and supervisory processes by which this treatment is provided. A major criterion for acceptance of manuscripts is the clinical significance of the subject matter. Manuscripts may take one of three forms: articles, reports, or letters.

Journal of Speech and Hearing Research

Year of Origin: 1958
Publisher: American Speech-Language-Hearing Assoc., 10801 Rockville Pike, Rockville, Maryland 20852. Tel: 301 897 5700
Editor: Tanya M. Gallagher
Subscription Rate: $45 one-year USA, $48 one-year Foreign
Circulation/Frequency: 43,000/Quarterly
Pages per Issue: 160
Author Payment: $65 page charge to author
Photo Policy: Camera Ready Accepted
Writer's Guidelines: American Psychological Association Style Manual
Scope of Journal: This journal pertains broadly to studies of the processes and disorders of speech, hearing, and language. Manuscripts may take the form of experimental reports—theoretical, tutorial, or review papers, brief research notes describing a procedure or instrumentation, and letters to the editor.

Journal of Studies on Alcohol

Year of Origin: 1940
Publisher: Rutgers Center of Alcohol Studies, P.O. Box 969, Piscataway, New Jersey 08854. Tel: 201 932 3510
Editor: Mark Keller, Acting Editor
Subscription Rate: $75 one-year USA, $85 one-year Foreign, $140 two-year USA, $160 two-year Foreign, $200 three-year USA, $230 three-year Foreign
Circulation/Frequency: 3,800/Monthly
Pages per Issue: Variable
Author Payment: None
Photo Policy: Black and White Glossies
Scope of Journal: This journal publishes in two parts: original articles of new research on all aspects of alcohol and alcohol problems and book reviews appear in odd-numbered months; abstracts and bibliography of current literature and subject and author indexes appear in even-numbered months.

Journal of Teacher Education

Year of Origin: 1950
Publisher: American Association of Colleges for Teacher Education, One Dupont Circle, Suite 610, Washington, D. C. 20036. Tel: 202 293 2450
Editor: Dr. Martin Haberman, Dean, Division of Urban Outreach, University of Wisconsin, Milwaukee, Wisconsin 53211. Tel: 414 963 5930
Subscription Rate: $25 one year
Circulation/Frequency: 6,500/six yearly
Pages per Issue: 64
Author Payment: 100% contributed
Photo Policy: Photos Not Accepted
Scope of Journal: This journal includes articles and papers dealing

with current, scholarly issues and research in teacher education today. Book reviews are included. Five of the six issues yearly carry themes. Refereed acceptance.

The Journal of Thoracic and Cardiovascular Surgery
Year of Origin: 1931
Publisher: The C. V. Mosby Company, 11830 Westline Industrial Drive, St. Louis, Missouri 83141. Tel: 314 872 8370
Editor: Dwight C. Mc Goon, MD, 200 First Street, SW, Rochester, Minnesota 55905. Tel: 507 284 8553
Subscription Rate: $72.00 one-year Institution USA, $87.25 International, $51.00 one-year Individual USA, $66.25 International, $40.80 one-year Student USA, $56.05 International
Circulation/Frequency: 10,760/Monthly
Pages per Issue: 170
Author Payment: None
Photo Policy: Black and White Glossies
Scope of Journal: This journal represents: The American Association for Thoracic Surgery, The Samson Thoracic Surgical Society. Articles submitted for publication should represent original communications related to the title and submitted exclusively to this journal.

Journal of Tropical Medicine and Hygiene
Publisher: Blackwell Scientific Publications Ltd, 8 John Street, London WC1N 2ES, England
Editor: Professor D. J. Bradley, Keppel Street, London WC1E 7HT, England
Subscription Rate: $75 one-year USA & Canada
Circulation/Frequency: 288/6 yearly
Pages per issue: about 65

Author Payment: None
Photo Policy: Black and White Glossies Accepted
Writer's Guidelines: Contact Editor
Scope of Journal: This journal covers all aspects of modern diagnosis and treatment in the field of tropical medicine . . . drawing on the disciplines of immunology, haematology, parasitology, etc.; the journal presents a multidisciplinary approach to the subject. Editorial emphasis is on community health, epidemiology and preventive medicine.

Journal of Urology
Year of Origin: 1917
Publisher: Williams and Wilkins Company, 428 East Preston Street, Baltimore, Maryland 21202. Tel: 301 528 4000
Editor: Herbert Brendler, M.D.
Subscription Rate: $90 one-year
Circulation/Frequency: 16,000/monthly
Pages per Issue: 200
Author Payment: None
Photo Policy: Black and White Glossies
Writer's Guidelines: Contact Editor
Scope of Journal: This journal considers articles in the area of urology for three sections: Clinical, Investigative, and survey.

Journal of Youth and Adolescence
Year of Origin: 1972
Publisher: Plenum Publishing Company, 233 Spring Street, New York, New York 10013. Tel: 212 620 8466
Editor: Daniel Offer
Subscription Rate: $110 one-year USA, $124 one-year foreign
Circulation/Frequency: 916/Bimonthly
Pages per Issue: 100–120
Author Payment: None
Photo Policy: large black and white glossies
Scope of Journal: Publishes an array

of articles pertinent to students and professionals in health and child education. Articles range from theoretical to actual case studies. High-level medium of communication for psychiatrists, psychologists, biologists, sociologists, educators, and other health professionals who address themselves to the subject of youth and adolescence.

Laboratory Medicine
Year of Origin: 1969
Publisher: American Society of Clinical Pathologists, 2100 West Harrison, Chicago, Illinois 60612. Tel. 312 738 1336
Editor: Elmer W. Koneman, M.D., Sandra M. Williamson (Managing Editor)
Subscription Rate: $22 one-year Individual USA, $25 one-year Institution USA, $30 one-year Individual Foreign, $33 one-year Institution Foreign, $3 single copy
Circulation/Frequency: Unavailable/Monthly
Pages per Issue: about 65
Author Payment: None
Photo Policy: Black and White Glossies at least 5 × 7
Scope of Journal: This journal welcomes articles from readers for publication. Education-oriented and technical topics related to the clinical laboratory will be considered. Extensive bibliographies and references are not recommended, but authors are requested to document fully their sources of reference.

Language, Speech, and Hearing Services in Schools
Year of Origin: 1970
Publisher: American Speech-Language-Hearing Assoc., 10801 Rockville Pike, Rockville, Maryland 20852. Tel: 301 897 5700

Editor: Patricia A. Broen
Subscription Rate: $20 one-year USA, $23 one-year Foreign
Circulation/Frequency: 43,000/Quarterly
Pages per Issue: 64–72
Author Payment: $50 page charge to author
Photo Policy: Camera Ready Accepted
Writer's Guidelines: American Psychological Association Style Manual
Scope of Journal: This journal pertains to speech, hearing, and language services for children, particularly in schools. Manuscripts deal with all aspects of clinical services to children including: nature, assessment and remediation of speech, hearing, and language disorders, program organization, management and supervision, and scholarly discussion of philosophical issues relating to school programming.

Law and Medicine and Health Care
Year of Origin: 1981
Publisher: American Society of Law and Medicine, 765 Commonwealth Avenue, 16th Floor, Boston, Massachusetts 02215. Tel: 617 262 4990
Editor: Miles J. Zaremski, JD, A. Edward Boudera, JD
Subscription Rate: $30 one-year
Circulation/Frequency: 5,000/6 yearly
Pages per Issue: 50
Author Payment: None
Photo Policy: Black and White Glossies
Scope of Journal: Original manuscripts are welcome dealing with current or emerging issues or problems in health law or medicolegal relations. Acceptable subject areas include: health law and policy; the legal aspects of medical practice; medical malpractice; nursing law and ethics; compensation medicine; risk manage-

ment; or any other interrelationships between law, medicine, and health care.

Man and His Environment . . . Journal of Environmental Systems
Year of Origin: 1983
Publisher: Baywood Publishing Company, Inc., 120 Marine Street, Box D, Farmingdale, New York 11735. Tel: 516 249 2464
Editor: Paul R. De Cicco
Subscription Rate: $27 one-year Individual, $51 one-year Institution (add $3 postage USA/Canada and add $7 postage elsewhere)
Circulation/Frequency: Unavailable/4 yearly
Pages per Issue: 70
Author Payment: Lead Author Receives Complimentary Copies of Issue + 20 Free Reprints
Photo Policy: Black and White Glossies
Scope of Journal: This journal deals with the recognition and solution of problems which relate to the system-complexes making up our total environment. Areas of major interest: environmental values and policy, decision making in shaping and management of environment, environment impact and land use, human behavior and the environment, air, land, and water pollution control, new technological applications to environmental problems and socio-economic interfaces with the environment.

Marriage and Family Review
Year of Origin: 1977
Publisher: Haworth Publishing Company, 28 East 22nd Street, New York, New York 10010. Tel: 212 228 2800
Editor: Marvin B. Sussman Unidel, Professor of Individual & Family Studies, College of Human Research,

University of Delaware, Newark, Delaware 19711
Subscription Rate: $36 one-year Individual, $48 one-year Institution, $75 one-year Library
Circulation/Frequency: 2,750/Quarterly
Pages per Issue: Variable
Author Payment: None
Photo Policy: Photos Not Accepted
Writer's Guidelines: Contact Editor
Scope of Journal: A thematic journal with each issue covering a single topic in the marriage and family field . . . includes reviews of recent literature. The editorial board consists of outstanding leaders in the field guaranteeing high standards that guide its editorial policies.

Maternal-Child Nursing Journal
Year of Origin: 1971
Publisher: University of Pittsburg, School of Nursing, 437 Victoria Hall, 3500 Victoria Street, Pittsburgh, Pennsylvania 15261. Tel: 412 624 3845
Editor: Corinne Barnes, Olive Rich
Subscription Rate: $12 one-year USA, $15 one-year Canada, $17 one-year Foreign, $4 single copies
Circulation/Frequency: 1,400/Quarterly
Pages per Issue: 60–80
Author Payment: None
Photo Policy: Black and White Glossies, 5 × 7
Scope of Journal: This journal is designed to serve the expert nurse practitioner in the care of mothers and children as a medium of exchange and stimulation in the furtherance of professional knowledge and competence. Articles, case studies, literature reviews, or reports of original research focused on patients and their nursing care are invited; also contains book reviews.

Media and Methods
Year of Origin: 1964
Publisher: American Society of Educators, 1511 Walnut Street, Philadelphia, Pennsylvania 19102. Tel: 215 563 3501
Editor: Ann Capputo
Subscription Rate: $24 one-year
Circulation/Frequency:
30,000/Monthly
Pages per Issue: 32–50
Author Payment: Subscription Provided
Photo Policy: Black and White Glossies Accepted
Scope of Journal: This journal publishes articles, resources, reviews, and information geared toward teachers, librarians and media specialists at the secondary and college level; practical information on combining a wide range of technologies with instructional practices in schools; articles on special education and mainstreaming periodically.

Medical Clinics of North America
Year of Origin: 1916
Publisher: W. B. Saunders, West Washington Square, Philadelphia, Pennsylvania 19105. Tel: 215 574 4700
Editor: Guest Editor For Each Issue
Subscription Rate: $33 one-year
Circulation/Frequency:
Unavailable/Bi-monthly
Pages per Issue: about 250
Author Payment: None
Photo Policy: Black and White Glossies
Scope of Journal: Hard cover periodical. Each issue is focused on a specific topic and contains 10 to 15 state-of-the-art reviews on current practice by leading specialists in the field. Unsolicited articles are not accepted. The "guest editor" of each is-

sue invites papers on areas of current interest.

Medical Economics
Year of Origin: 1923
Publisher: Thomas J. McGill, Medical Economics Company, 680 Kinderkamack Road, Oradell, New Jersey 07649. Tel: 201 262 3030
Editor: Don L. Berg
Subscription Rate: $44 one year
Circulation/Frequency:
167,000/Bimonthly
Pages per Issue: 180–300
Author Payment: 30% contributed; typical payment $200 for 1,500–2,000 word manuscript
Photo Policy: 8 × 10 black and white glossies or 35 mm transparencies
Scope of Journal: This journal publishes non-clinical articles dealing with: practice management, patient relations, sociomedical issues, medicolegal issues, personal finance.

Medical Education
Publisher: Blackwell Scientific Publications Ltd., Osney Mead, Oxford, OX 2 OEL, England. Tel: 0865 40201
Editor: H. J. Walton, 9 Forrest Road, Edinburgh, EH1 2QH, Scotland
Subscription Rate: $120 one-year USA & Canada
Circulation/Frequency: 1,810/6 yearly
Pages per Issue: about 75
Author Payment: None
Photo Policy: Black and White Glossies Accepted
Writer's Guidelines: Contact Editor
Scope of Journal: All topical issues of students in medical fields both undergraduate and postgraduate. Included are: selection of entrants, teaching methods, assessment techniques, curriculum reforms, and the training of medical teachers.

**Medical Letter on Drugs &
Therapeutics**
Year of Origin: 1959
Publisher: Medical Letter, Inc., 56
Harrison Street, New Rochelle, New
York 10801. Tel: 914 235 0500
Editor: Mark Abramowicz, M. D.
Subscription Rate: $24.50 one-year,
$12.25 one-year students
Circulation/Frequency: 160,000/16
yearly
Pages per Issue: about 4
Author Payment: None
Photo Policy: Photos Not Accepted
Writer's Guidelines: Use Format
Within Letter
Scope of Journal: This letter includes
evaluation of new therapeutic drugs
or reevaluation of old drugs and oc-
casionally deals with drugs for
specific diseases.

Medical World News
Year of Origin: 1971
Publisher: HEI Publishing Company,
Inc., 211 East 43rd Street, New York,
New York 10017. Tel: 212 490 7801
Editor: Larry Frederick
Subscription Rate: $30 one-year
Circulation/Frequency:
118,000/Bimonthly
Pages per Issue: 96 average
Author Payment: Upon acceptance
$70/per 500 words
Photo Policy: Photos of all kinds accepted
Scope of Journal: This journal reports on all significant developments
in both the practice and science of
medicine throughout the world. Emphasis on new clinical research that
could or should change medical practice. Not interested in local events,
updates, overviews, personality features, personnel or fund-raising announcements, building expansions,
annual reports, etc.

Mental Retardation
Year of Origin: 1963
Publisher: American Association on
Mental Deficiency, 5101 Wisconsin
Avenue NW, Washington D. C.
20016. Tel: 202 686 5400
Editor: Reginald Jones, PhD, Institute
of Human Development, 1208 Tol-
man Hall, University of California,
Berkeley, California 94720
Subscription Rate: $26 one-year
Circulation/Frequency: 12,500
Pages per Issue: 64 average
Author Payment: None
Photo Policy: Release Required
Scope of Journal: This journal attempts to meet the needs of therapists, administrators, and advocates
for information about effective ways
to help retarded people. Thus, new
teaching approaches, administrative
tools, criticisms, and case studies are
welcome as are research studies that
emphasize the application of new
methods. Philosophical essays and
satirical pieces are also welcome if
they are well-expressed, stimulating,
and in good taste.

Merrill-Palmer Quarterly
Year of Origin: 1954
Publisher: Wayne State University
Press, 5959 Woodward, Detroit,
Michigan 48202. Tel: 313 577 4603
Editor: Carolyn U. Shantz, Editor, Eli
Saltz, Associate Editor, Department of
Psychology, Wayne State University,
Detroit, Michigan 48202. Tel: 313
577 4603
Subscription Rate: $20 one-year Indi-
vidual, $36 two-year Individual, $50
three-year Individual
Circulation/Frequency: 1,800/Quar-
terly
Pages per Issue: about 130
Author Payment: None
Photo Policy: Black and White Glos-
sies

Scope of Journal: This journal publishes empirical studies, theoretical articles, and reviews of the literature dealing with the development of infants, children, and adolescents; occasionally commentaries on major articles and book reviews.

Milbank Memorial Fund Quarterly/ Health and Society
Year of Origin: 1923
Publisher: The MIT Press, 28 Carleton Street, Cambridge, Massachusetts 02142. Tel: 617 253 2889
Editor: David P. Willis, 1 East 7th Street, New York, New York 10021. Tel: 210 570 4807
Subscription Rate: $20 one-year Individual, $42 one-year Institution
Circulation/Frequency: 3,000/Quarterly
Pages per Issue: 180
Author Payment: 100% contributed
Photo Policy: Photos Not Accepted
Scope of Journal: Publishes articles on history, development, and analysis of health policy from social sciences, economics, history, and health services research. Articles may be based on empirical research or policy analysis; rigor and clarity are essential.

Modern Concepts of Cardiovascular Disease
Year of Origin: 1930
Publisher: American Heart Association, 7320 Greenville Avenue, Dallas, Texas 75231. Tel: 214 750 5300
Editor: Frank I. Marcus, MD
Subscription Rate: Binders holding two years' issues $2.50, Bound two years' issues $5
Circulation/Frequency: 100,000/Monthly
Pages per Issue: Leaflet
Author Payment: None
Photo Policy: Photos Not Accepted
Writer's Guidelines: Contact Editor

Scope of Journal: A concise monthly review of one cardiovascular subject.

Modern Health Care
Year of Origin: 1974
Publisher: Crain Communications, Inc.; 740 North Rush Street, Chicago, Illinois 60611. Tel: 312 649 5200
Editor: Donald Johnson
Subscription Rate: $35 one-year
Circulation/Frequency: Unavailable/Monthly
Pages per Issue: 200–250
Author Payment: None
Photo Policy: Black and White Glossies
Writer's Guidelines: Contact Editor
Scope of Journal: This is a business-oriented journal for health care providers and publishes an array of articles dealing with administration, reimbursement, law, legislation and marketing.

National Intravenous Therapy Association
Year of Origin: 1978
Publisher: J. B. Lippincott Company, East Washington Square, Philadelphia, Pennsylvania 19105. Tel: 215 574
Editor: Mary Larkin, R. N., 93 Concord Avenue, Suite 4, Belmont, Massachusetts 02178. Tel: 617 489 2947
Subscription Rate: $31 one-year Individual USA, $35 one-year Individual Foreign
Circulation/Frequency: 1,600/Monthly
Pages per Issue: 50–70
Author Payment: None
Photo Policy: Black and White Glossies
Scope of Journal: This journal is the official publication of the National Intravenous Therapy Association and is published to provide and promote communication among all persons professionally involved in the field of

intravenous therapy. It welcomes manuscripts relevant to the above theme and encourages submissions from readers.

The Nation's Health
Year of Origin: 1970
Publisher: American Public Health Association, 1015 Fifteenth Street NW, Washington D. C. 20005. Tel: 202 789 5664
Editor: Kathryn Foxhole
Subscription Rate: $8 USA, $10 Foreign, $1 Single Copy
Circulation/Frequency: International/Monthly
Pages per Issue: 12–16
Author Payment: None
Photo Policy: Black and White Glossies
Writer's Guidelines: Contact Editor
Scope of Journal: This publication is a monthly newspaper on public health issues and policies. It includes national public health items regarding legislation, regulations, and developments; also includes business of the American Public Health Association.

New England Journal of Medicine
Year of Origin: 1928
Publisher: Massachusetts Medical Society, 1172 Commonwealth Avenue, Boston, Massachusetts 02134. Tel: 617 734 9800
Editor: Arnold S. Relman, MD, 10 Shattuck Street, Boston, Massachusetts 02115
Subscription Rate: $48 one-year USA Individual, $58 one-year Canada Individual, $66 one-year Foreign Individual, $30 one-year USA Student, $40 one-year Canada Student, $50 one-year Foreign Student
Circulation/Frequency: 206,886/Weekly
Pages per Issue: 60–80

Author Payment: None
Photo Policy: Photos Not Accepted
Scope of Journal: This is a general medical journal which presents original articles and interpretive reviews of new developments in the major aspects of medicine: its science, its art and practice, and its position in today's social-political structure.

Nurse Educator
Year of Origin: 1915
Publisher: Nursing Resources, 12 Lakeside Park, 607 North Avenue, Wakefield, Massachusetts 01880. Tel: 617 246 3130
Editor: John W. Watkins, Donna Peltz, Asst. Editor
Subscription Rate: $15 one-year Individual, $30 one-year Institution
Circulation/Frequency: 18,500/Bimonthly, (additional Issue in November)
Pages per Issue: 20
Author Payment: None
Photo Policy: Photos Not Accepted
Scope of Journal: The objective of this journal is to provide a high level source of information on both the practical and theoretical aspects of nursing education, including educational philosophy, curriculum and program development, teaching methods, instructional materials, testing and measurement, and administration.

Nursing Clinics of North America
Year of Origin: 1966
Publisher: W. B. Saunders, West Washington Square, Philadelphia, Pennsylvania 19105. Tel: 215 574 4700
Editor: Guest Editor For Each Issue
Subscription Rate: $20 one-year
Circulation/Frequency: Unavailable/Quarterly
Pages per Issue: about 250

Author Payment: None
Photo Policy: Black and White Glossies
Scope of Journal: Hard cover periodical. Each issue is focused on a specific topic and contains 10 to 15 state-of-the-art reviews on current clinical practice by leading specialists in the field. Unsolicited articles are not accepted. The "guest editor" of each issue invites papers on areas of current interest.

Nursing Journal
Year of Origin: 1908
Publisher: Nurses' Association Inc., Box 2128, Wellington, New Zealand. Tel: 04-850 847
Editor: Ann Cherrington
Subscription Rate: $15 one-year USA
Circulation/Frequency: 14,777/monthly
Pages per Issue: 32–40
Author Payment: 60% contributed
Photo Policy: Black and White Glossies
Scope of Journal: Material is welcome for any section of the journal—letters to the editor, articles relating to any area of nursing, reports of study days, seminars, etc. news and events.

Nursing Leadership
Year of Origin: 1977
Publisher: Charles B. Slack, Inc., 6900 Grove Road, Thorofare, New Jersey, 08086. Tel: 609 848 1000
Editor: Dorothy F. Corona, RN
Subscription Rate: $14 one-year
Circulation/Frequency: 2,047/Quarterly
Pages per Issue: 36
Author Payment: None
Photo Policy: Black and White Glossies
Scope of Journal: Original articles pertaining to all levels of leadership in nursing.

Nursing Management
Year of Origin: 1970
Publisher: Nursing Management, 3734 Glenway Avenue, Cincinnati, Ohio 45205. Tel: 513 251 4335
Editor: Leah L. Curtin
Subscription Rate: $18 one-year
Circulation/Frequency: 85,000/Monthly
Pages per Issue: 70–90
Author Payment: None
Photo Policy: Black and White Glossies
Scope of Journal: The major focus of this journal is mid-level management issues, problems, activities, etc. Also covered are important political, social and professional viewpoints.

Nursing Mirror
Year of Origin: 1895
Publisher: Surrey House, Throwsley Way, Sutton, Surrey, England
Editor: T. Brock and Mark Allen
Subscription Rate: $162 one-year airmail, $91 one-year regular mail
Circulation/Frequency: 50,000/Weekly
Pages per Issue: 58
Author Payment: Approximately $55 per 750–1,000 words
Photo Policy: Accepted By Negotiation
Writer's Guidelines: Contact Editor
Scope of Journal: Wide range of nursing care articles from Science K Post-Basic training procedures; also includes articles management and patient care histories.

Nursing News, (previously Christian Nurse)
Year of Origin: 1964 (previously 1931)
Publisher: Christian Medical Association of India, Council Lodge, P.B. 24, Nagpur 440 001
Editor: Miss Sigamoni
Subscription Rate: $10 one-year

Circulation/Frequency:
2,000/Bi-monthly
Pages per Issue: 35–40
Author Payment: None
Photo Policy: Photos Not Accepted
Writer's Guidelines: Contact Editor
Scope of Journal: This journal is the official publication of the Nurses League of the Medical Association of India. It contains professional scientific articles, news, reports of regional activities of the League. The membership is from big teaching hospitals to primary health centers. Membership is from all around the world (USA, England, Canada, Arabia, and Persia).

Nursing Outlook
Year of Origin: 1953
Publisher: American Journal of Nursing Company, 555 West 57th Street, New York, New York 10019. Tel: 212 582 8820.
Editor: Lucie S. Kelly, RN
Subscription Rate: $22 one-year USA, $41 one-year Canada, $34 one-year Foreign, $41 two-year USA, $61 two-year Canada, $65 two-year Foreign
Circulation/Frequency:
21,000/Bimonthly
Pages per Issue: 72 average
Author Payment: None
Photo Policy: Black and White Glossies
Scope of Journal: A Broadly based nonclinical journal; the purpose is to contribute to the growth of nursing and related health professions, and knowledge base by presenting a diversity of ideas on professional trends, concepts in nursing education, administration, community health, and nontraditional nursing roles.

Nursing Research
Year of Origin: 1952
Publisher: American Journal of Nursing Company, 555 West 57th Street, New York, New York 10019. Tel: 212 582 8820
Editor: Florence Downs, Ed.D./ F.A.A.N. Tel: 215 898 8286
Subscription Rate: $23 one-year Individual USA, $35 one-year Institution USA
Circulation/Frequency:
9,000/Bi-monthly
Pages per Issue: 63
Author Payment: None
Photo Policy: Black and White Glossies
Scope of Journal: This journal will consider articles for publication that have to do with research that advances nursing science; also, theoretical position papers are included. The official journal of the American Nurses' Association.

Nursing Times
Publisher: Macmillan Journals Ltd., 4 Little Essex Street, London WC2R 3LF. Tel: 836 1776
Editor: Alison Dunn
Subscription Rate: $85 one-year USA, £28 one-year UK
Circulation/Frequency: 1,200/Weekly
Pages per Issue: 44 edited pages
Author Payment: £50 per article
Photo Policy: Photos Not Accepted
Scope of Journal: A weekly publication covering all aspects of nursing practice, education and management. Includes news and current affairs, nursing care studies, clinical articles, general feature articles, and teaching aids; also covers readers' letters and other information features.

Nutrition News
Year of Origin: 1937
Publisher: National Dairy Council, 6300 North River Road, Rosemont, Illinois 60018. Tel: 312 696 1020
Editor: Dusty Rhoades, 600 Old Barn

Road, Barrington, Illinois 60010. Tel: 312 382 1833
Subscription Rate: $10 one-year
Circulation/Frequency: 77,700/4 yearly
Pages per Issue: 4–6
Author Payment: None
Photo Policy: Black and White Glossies
Writer's Guidelines: Contact Editor; No Unsolicited Articles
Scope of Journal: This newsletter is intended for those who are interested in practical applications of nutrition information but who might not be in a position to follow closely the more technical developments in food and nutrition research. The lead article features a current topic in nutrition. Other articles report health and nutrition education activities carried on in a wide variety of professional, educational and business/industry groups.

Nutrition Reviews
Year of Origin: 1979
Publisher: The Nutrition Foundation, Inc.
Editor: Dr. Robert E. Olson, MD, Dept. of Biochemistry, St. Louis University, School of Medicine, 1402 South Grand, St. Louis, Missouri 63104. Tel: 314 664 9800, ext. 174
Subscription Rate: $20 one-year Individual, $10 one-year Student, $36 two-year Individual
Circulation/Frequency: 8,000/Monthly
Pages per Issue: 32
Author Payment: 10¢ a word
Photo Policy: 5 × 7 Black and White Glossies
Scope of Journal: This journal aims to keep professionally trained people abreast of current progress in nutrition, and to have available an unbiased, authoritative review of its research literature. This journal also publishes case reports; book notices, special reports and meeting announcements.

Nutrition Today
Year of Origin: 1966
Publisher: Nutrition Today, Inc., 703 Giddings Avenue, Annapolis, Maryland 21401. Tel: 301 267 8616
Editor: Cortez F. Enloe, Jr., MD
Subscription Rate: $17.75 USA/ Canada, $21.75 Foreign
Circulation/Frequency: 20,000/Bimonthly
Pages per Issue: 40
Author Payment: None
Photo Policy: Black and White Glossies
Scope of Journal: This journal is dedicated to the increase and dissemination of nutritional knowledge.

Occupational Health
Year of Origin: 1949
Publisher: Occupational Health, 10 Greycoat Place, London SW1P 1SB, UK. Tel: 01 222 7191
Editor: Michael Bangs
Subscription Rate: $45 one-year
Circulation/Frequency: 3,700/Monthly
Pages per Issue: 48–56
Author Payment: By Agreement
Photo Policy: Prints & Transparencies Accepted
Scope of Journal: Aimed primarily at occupational health care professionals; also covers industrial safety.

Occupational Health Nursing
Year of Origin: 1950
Publisher: Charles B. Slack, Inc., 6900 Grove Road, Thorofare, New Jersey 08086. Tel: 848 1000
Editor: Margaret Carnine, RN
Subscription Rate: $17 one-year
Circulation/Frequency: 13,564/Monthly
Pages per Issue: 52
Author Payment: None

Photo Policy: Black and White Glossies
Writer's Guidelines: Contact Publisher
Scope of Journal: Original articles of interest to occupational health nurses and other members of the occupational health team.

Occupational Therapy in Mental Health
Year of Origin: 1980
Publisher: Haworth Publishing Company, 28 East 22nd Street, New York, New York 10010. Tel: 212 228 2800
Editor: Diane Maslen, Director, Activities Therapy, Sheppard and Enoch Pratt Hospital, North Charles Street, Baltimore, Maryland 21204
Subscription Rate: $28 one-year Individual, $48 one-year Institution, $65 one-year Library
Circulation/Frequency: 2,100/Quarterly
Pages Per Issue: Variable
Author Payment: None
Photo Policy: Photos Not Accepted
Writer's Guidelines: Contact Editor
Scope of Journal: The only journal focusing on the help available from Occupational Therapy services in both community programs and psychiatric hospitals. All aspects of psychosocial occupational therapy are explored indepth.

Omega: Journal of Death and Dying
Year of Origin: 1970
Publisher: Baywood Publishing Company, Inc., 120 Marine Street, Box D, Farmingdale, New York 11735. Tel: 516 249 2464
Editor: Robert J. Kastenbaum
Subscription Rate: $27 one-year Individual, $51 one-year Institution, (Add $3 postage in USA/Canada and Add $7 postage elsewhere)
Circulation/Frequency: 1200/4 yearly

Pages per Issue: 135
Author Payment: Lead Author Receives Complimentary Copies of Issue + 20 Free Reprints
Photo Policy: Black and White Glossies
Scope of Journal: This journal draws significant contributions from such diverse fields as psychology, sociology, law, anthropology, medicine, education, history, and literature. Every aspect of this universal subject is explored: terminal illness; suicide; violence and disaster; values; concepts and attitudes about death, bereavement, and grief. It is an excellent classroom supplement as well as a reliable guide for clinicians and health professionals.

Ophthalmic Surgery
Year of Origin: 1969
Publisher: Charles B. Slack, Inc., 6900 Grove Road, Thorofare, New Jersey 08086. Tel: 609 848 1000
Editor: George W. Weinstein, MD
Subscription Rate: $45 one-year
Circulation/Frequency: 12,924/Monthly
Pages per Issue: 100
Author Payment: None
Photo Policy: Black and White Glossies
Scope of Journal: Publishes original articles of interest to ophthalmologists and ophthalmic surgeons.

Ophthalmology
Year of Origin: 1907
Publisher: J. B. Lippincott Company, East Washington Square, Philadelphia, Pennsylvania 19105. Tel: 215 574 4216
Editor: Paul Henkind, MD, Ph.D.
Subscription Rate: $60 one-year Individual USA, $78 one-year Institution Foreign
Circulation/Frequency:

14,011/Monthly
Pages per Issue: 80–100
Author Payment: None
Photo Policy: Black and White Glossies, (Colored at Author's Expense)
Writer's Guidelines: Contact Publisher
Scope of Journal: Acceptance of papers for the program of the American Academy of Ophthalmology or of original unsolicited contributions pertaining to clinical, basic, or educational aspects of ophthalmology. Assurance must be given that these papers have not been previously published.

Oral Surgery, Oral Medicine, Oral Pathology

Year of Origin: 1948
Publisher: The C. V. Mosby Company, 11830 Westline Industrial Drive, St. Louis, Missouri 63141. Tel: 314 872 8370
Editor: Dr. Robert B. Shira, Dean, School of Dental Medicine, Tufts University, Kneeland Street, Boston, Massachusetts 02111
Subscription Rate: $51.50 one-year Institution USA, $63 International, $30.50 one-year Individual USA, $42 International, $24.40 one-year Student USA, $35.90 International
Circulation/Frequency: 12,530/Monthly
Pages per Issue: 120
Author Payment: None
Photo Policy: Black and White Glossies
Scope of Journal: An official journal of Americal Academy of Oral Pathology; American Institute of Oral Biology; American Academy of Dental Radiology; American College of Stomatologic Surgeons; Organization of Teachers of Oral Diagnosis and state associations. Articles submitted for publication should represent original communications related to the title and submitted exclusively to this journal.

Orthopedic Clinics of North America

Year of Origin: 1970
Publisher: W. B. Saunders, West Washington Square. Philadelphia, Pennsylvania 19105. Tel: 215 574 4700
Editor: Guest Editor for Each Issue
Subscription Rate: $38 one-year
Circulation/Frequency: Unavailable/Quarterly
Pages per Issue: about 250
Author Payment: None
Photo Policy: Black and White Glossies
Scope of Journal: Hard cover periodical. Each issue is focused on a specific topic and contains 10 to 15 state-of-the-art reviews on current clinical practice by leading specialists in the field. Unsolicited articles are not accepted. The "guest editor" of each issue invites papers on areas of current interest.

Orthopedics

Year of Origin: 1978
Publisher: Charles B. Slack, Inc., 6900 Grove Road, Thorofare, New Jersey 08086. Tel: 609 848 1000
Editor: H. Andrew Wissinger, MD
Subscription Rate: $45 one-year
Circulation/Frequency: 23,000/Monthly
Pages per Issue: 120 average
Author Payment: None
Photo Policy: Black and White Glossies or Color Prints (5 × 7 preferred)
Scope of Journal: This journal publishes reports or original research and case reports as well as departments addressing particular aspects of orthopedics, radiology, book reviews, products and developments, and general news pertinent to orthopedics.

Orthopedics Today
Year of Origin: 1981
Publisher: Charles B. Slack, Inc.,
6900 Grove Road, Thorofare, New
Jersey 08086
Editor: Eric Baloff
Subscription Rate: $35 one-year
Circulation/Frequency:
24,000/Monthly
Pages per Issue: 32–36
Author Payment: None
Photo Policy: Black and White Glossies or Color Slides okay (5 × 7 preferred)
Scope of Journal: This journal disseminates timely information to the community of orthopedic specialists. Each issue contains reports of recent meetings, including new techniques and advances in orthopedic treatment. Featured columns discuss new developments in tax laws, guidance for investment opportunities, and legal aspects of a physician's practice. Sections include introductions of new products, lists of meetings and educational opportunities, book reviews, and legislative news.

Otolaryngologic Clinics of North America
Year of Origin: 1968
Publisher: W. B. Saunders, West Washington Square, Philadelphia, Pennsylvania 19105. Tel: 215 574 4700
Editor: Guest Editor For Each Issue
Subscription Rate: $44 one-year
Circulation/Frequency:
Unavailable/Quarterly
Pages per Issue: about 250
Author Payment: None
Photo Policy: Black and White Glossies
Scope of Journal: Hard cover periodical. Each issue is focused on a specific topic and contains 10 to 15 state-of-the art reviews on current clinical practice by leading specialists in the field. Unsolicited articles are not accepted. The "guest editor" of each issue invites papers on areas of current interest.

Parasite Immunology
Publisher: Blackwell Scientific Publications Ltd., 8 John Street, London WC1N 2ES
Editor: T. J. Terry, G. A. T. Targett, 8 John Street, London SC1N 2ES
Subscription Rate: £60 one-year UK, £72 one-year Overseas, $165 one-year USA/Canada
Circulation/Frequency: 420/Bi-monthly
Pages per Issue: about 20
Author Payment: None
Photo Policy: Black and White Glossies
Writer's Guidelines: Contact Editor
Scope of Journal: This journal is devoted to research on parasite immunology in the widest sense. Emphasis is placed on new hosts control parasites, and the immuno pathological reaction which takes place in the course of parasitic infection. This publication welcomes original work.

Patient Care
Year of Origin: 1967
Publisher: Patient Care Communications, Inc., 16 Thorndal Circle, Box 1245, Darien, Connecticut 06820, (John A. Krieger)
Editor: Clayton Raker Hasser
Subscription Rate: $42 one-year USA, $50 one-year Canada, $70 one-year Foreign
Circulation/Frequency: 108,000/21 yearly
Pages per Issue: 125–300
Author Payment: Free-lance articles on assignment only
Photo Policy: On assignment only
Writer's Guidelines: Editor Contact

Scope of Journal: Material published is devoted to diagnosis, treatment, and long-term management related to specific symptoms and complaints. Other inclusions are: management medicine, any factor that impinges on patients' satisfaction with appropriate use of the services available, Flow-charts—memory aids, Patient Education Aids, etc.

Patient Education and Counseling
Year of Origin: 1978
Publisher: Excerpta Medica, Box 3085, Princeton, New Jersey 08540. Tel: 609 896 9450
Editor: Peter Maguire, MD, Scott K. Simonds, Dr. P.H., Cyril M. Worby, MD
Subscription Rate: $20 one-year Individuals, $40 one-year Institutions
Circulation/Frequency: Unavailable/Quarterly
Pages per Issue: 55–60
Author Payment: None
Photo Policy: Photos Not Accepted
Writer's Guidelines: Contact Excerpta Medica
Scope of Journal: An international, interdisciplinary journal which seeks to achieve as broad a perspective as possible. Contributions deal with: role of the family and the different members of the health-care team, as well as with the impact on hospital and health-care organization on patient counselling and education. It attempts to determine ways counselling and patient education can be enhanced in these settings.

The Pavlovian Journal of Biological Science
Year of Origin: 1982
Publisher: J. B. Lippincott Company, East Washington Square, Philadelphia, Pennsylvania 19105. Tel: 215 574 4200
Editor: F. J. McGuigan, Performance Research Laboratory, University of Louisville, Louisville, Kentucky 40292
Subscription Rate: Contact Editor
Circulation/Frequency: New/Quarterly
Pages per Issue: Variable
Author Payment: None
Photo Policy: Black and White Glossies
Scope of Journal: This journal is a quarterly publication containing articles pertaining to empirical, theoretical, review, apparatus, and historical topics.

Pediatric Annals
Year of Origin: 1972
Publisher: Charles B. Slack, Inc., 6900 Grove Road, Thorofare, New Jersey 08086. Tel: 609 848 1000
Editor: Milton I. Levine, MD
Subscription Rate: $30 one-year
Circulation/Frequency: 26,300/Monthly
Pages per Issue: 60–75
Author Payment: None
Photo Policy: Photos Not Accepted
Writer's Guidelines: Contact Editor
Scope of Journal: The aim of this journal is to provide the pediatrician with new information on diagnosis and patient treatment that will be useful to him in his practice.

Pediatric Clinics of North America
Year of Origin: 1954
Publisher: W. B. Saunders, West Washington Square, Philadelphia, Pennsylvania 19105. Tel: 215 574 4700
Editor: Guest Editor For Each Issue
Subscription Rate: $30 one-year
Circulation/Frequency: Unavailable/Bi-monthly
Pages per Issue: about 250
Author Payment: None
Photo Policy: Black and White Glos-

sies
Scope of Journal: Hard cover periodical. Each issue is focused on a specific topic and contains 10 to 15 state-of-the-art reviews on current clinical practice by leading specialists in the field. Unsolicited articles are not accepted. The "guest editor" of each issue invites papers on areas of current interest.

Pediatric Nursing
Year of Origin: 1975
Publisher: Anthony J. Jannetti, Inc., North Woodbury Road, Box 56, Pittman, New Jersey 08071. Tel: 609 589 2319
Editor: Karen Mitchell
Subscription Rate: $15 one-year
Circulation/Frequency: 9,000/Bi-monthly
Pages per Issue: 70–80
Author Payment: None
Photo Policy: Black and White Glossies
Writer's Guidelines: Contact Editor
Scope of Journal: This publication is the official journal of the National Association of Pediatric Nurses, Associates, and Practitioners. It provides a forum for this vital segment of the health care industry and is a vehicle for clinical "how-to" editorials.

Perceptual and Motor Skills
Year of Origin: 1948
Publisher: R. B. Ammons, Box 9229, Missoula, Montana 59807
Editor: R. B. Ammons, C. H. Ammons
Subscription Rate: $122.60 one-year
Circulation/Frequency: International/Bi-monthly
Pages per Issue: 100–115
Author Payment: Author pays $27.50 per page, 50/200 free reprints/by pages
Photo Policy: Black and White Glos-

sies; 4½ × 6", Original Drawings
Scope of Journal: The purpose of this journal is to encourage scientific originality and creativity. Material of the following kinds is carried: experimental or theoretical articles dealing with perception or motor skills, especially as affected by experience; articles on general methodology; new material listing and reviews. An attempt is made to make the approach interdisciplinary.

Perspectives in Biology & Medicine
Year of Origin: 1957
Publisher: University of Chicago Press, 5801 South Ellis Avenue, Chicago, Illinois 60637. Tel: 312 962 7600
Editor: Richard L. Landua, MD
Subscription Rate: $20 one-year Individuals, $28 one-year Institutions
Circulation/Frequency: 4,500/Quarterly
Pages per Issue: 160
Author Payment: None
Photo Policy: Photos Not Accepted
Writer's Guidelines: Contact Editor
Scope of Journal: Publishes articles on a broad range of subjects with emphasis on essays in which medicine and basic biology are interrelated, and biomedical science is integrated with the humanities and social sciences.

Perspectives in Psychiatric Care
Year of Origin: 1963
Publisher: Nursing Publications, Inc., Box 218, Hillsdale, New Jersey 07642. Tel: 201 391 7845
Editor: Alice R. Clarke
Subscription Rate: $18 one-year Individual, $20 one-year Institution
Circulation/Frequency: 6,000/Quarterly
Pages per Issue: 40–60
Author Payment: None

Photo Policy: Black and White Glossies

Writer's Guidelines: Contact Editor

Scope of Journal: This is a specialty journal directed to psychiatric-mental health nurses and is clinical oriented. It includes areas such as education, administration, clinical practice, etc.

Phi Delta Kappan

Year of Origin: 1914
Publisher: Phi Delta Kappa, P.O. Box 689, Bloomington, Indiana 47402. Tel: 812 339 1156
Editor: Robert W. Cole, Jr.
Subscription Rate: $20 one year
Circulation/Frequency: 135,000/10 yearly
Pages per Issue: 72
Author Payment: None
Photo Policy: Some freelance photos used
Scope of Journal: This journal publishes articles concerned with educational research, service, and leadership; issues, trends, and policy are emphasized. Editors look for educational significance and readability.

Physical and Occupational Therapy in Geriatrics

Year of Origin: 1981
Publisher: The Haworth Press, 28 East 22nd Street, New York, New York 10010. Tel: 212 228 2800
Editor: Jean M. Kiernat, Center for Health Sciences, Occupational Therapy Program, 1300 University Avenue, Madison, Wisconsin 53706. Tel: 608 262 2936
Subscription Rate: $28 one-year $48 two-years, $65 three-years
Circulation/Frequency: 1,110/Quarterly
Pages per issue: 80–100
Author Payment: None
Photo Policy: Photos Not Accepted
Writer's Guidelines: Contact Editor

Scope of Journal: Publishes an array of articles, materials and announcements pertinent to Physical and Occupational Therapy in Geriatrics.

Physical and Occupational Therapy in Pediatrics

Year of Origin: 1980
Publisher: Haworth Press, 28 East 22nd Street, New York, New York 10010. Tel: 212 228 2800
Editor: Suzann Cambell, Department of Medical Allied Health Professions, University of North Carolina, Chapel Hill, North Carolina 27514. Tel: 919 966 3046
Subscription Rate: $28 one-year, $48 two-years, $65 three-years
Circulation/Frequency: 1,110/Quarterly
Pages per Issue: 85–90
Author Payment: None
Photo Policy: Photos Not Accepted
Writer's Guidelines: Contact Editor
Scope of Journal: Publishes an array of articles, materials and announcements pertinent to Physical and Occupational Therapy in Pediatrics.

Physiological Reviews

Year of Origin: 1921
Publisher: American Physiological Society, 9650 Rockville Pike, Bethesda, Maryland 20014. Tel: 301 530 7160
Editor: Stephen R. Geiger
Subscription Rate: $45 USA, $55 Foreign
Circulation/Frequency: Unavailable/Quarterly
Pages per Issue: about 250
Author Payment: None
Photo Policy: Black and White Glossies
Scope of Journal: The journal contains invited critical reviews of physiological topics as well as reviews in biochemistry, nutrition, general physiology, biophysics, and neuroscience.

Reviews are invited from the leading scientists worldwide by American Editorial Board and a European Editorial Committee.

The Physiologist
Year of Origin: 1887
Publisher: American Physiological Society, 9650 Rockville Pike, Bethesda, Maryland 20014. Tel: 301 530 7160
Editor: Stephen R. Geiger
Subscription Rate: $30 USA, $40 Foreign
Circulation/Frequency: Unavailable/Bimonthly
Pages per Issue: Variable
Author Payment: None
Photo Policy: Black and White Glossies
Scope of Journal: The Physiologist contains material not included in journals of primary publication but of interest to all physiologists: articles and vignettes on physiological history, educational approaches, teaching laboratory experiment protocols, announcements of national and international meetings, abstracts of papers presented at meetings, proceedings of symposia and specialty meetings, career opportunities, and reports of American Physiological Society affairs.

Plastic and Reconstructive Surgery
Year of Origin: 1946
Publisher: Williams and Wilkins Company, 428 East Preston Street, Baltimore, Maryland 21202. Tel: 301 528 4100
Editor: Dr. Robert M. Goldwyn
Subscription Rate: $70 one-year
Circulation/Frequency: Unavailable/Monthly
Pages per Issue: 150 average
Author Payment: None
Photo Policy: Black and White Glossies
Writer's Guidelines: Contact Editor

Scope of Journal: This journal publishes an array of articles and papers dealing with plastic and reconstructive surgery.

Point of View Magazine
Year of Origin: 1964
Publisher: Ethicon, Inc., Route 22, Somerville, New Jersey 08876
Editor: Lucy Jo Atkinson, RN
Subscription Rate: Free
Circulation/Frequency: 51,000/Quarterly
Pages per Issue: 23–25
Author Payment: No unsolicited articles
Photo Policy: Photos, Slides & Drawings Accepted
Writer's Guidelines: Contact Editor
Scope of Journal: Publishes articles and suggestions for hospital personnel; articles range from amusing to technical and includes advertisements and self-assessment quizes.

Population and Environment: Behavioral and Social Issues
Year of Origin: 1976
Publisher: Human Science Press, 72 Fifth Avenue, New York, New York 10011. Tel: 212 243 6000
Editor: Vaida D. Thompson, Ralph Taylor
Subscription Rate: $58 Institution, $25 Individual
Circulation/Frequency: 950/Quarterly
Pages per Issue: 64 average
Author Payment: None
Photo Policy: Black and White Glossies
Writer's Guidelines: No Specific Guidelines; Use Format Within Journal
Scope of Journal: This journal is devoted to the publication of scholarly, empirical and theoretical articles on population and environmental phenomena and issues from architec-

tural impacts to wilderness perception, from reproductive behavior to migration. While primary emphasis is a psychological treatment of population and environment, behavior phenomena, articles from other related disciplines also appear.

Postgraduate Medical Journal
Publisher: Blackwell Scientific Publications Ltd., Osney Mead, Oxford, OX 2 OLL
Editor: B. I. Hoffbrand, Archway Wing, Whittington Hospital, Archway, London N19 5NF
Subscription Rate: £52 one-year UK, £62.50 one-year Overseas, $137.50 one-year USA/Canada
Circulation/Frequency: 1,770/Monthly
Pages per Issue: 75
Author Payment: None
Photo Policy: Black and White Glossies
Writer's Guidelines: Contact Editor
Scope of Journal: Designed for all those who wish to keep abreast of the most important trends in clincal medicine. It is particularly useful for the young postgraduate and should form an integral part of their training; it also provides a medium for the publication of new work of clinical relevance.

Prevention in Human Services
Year of Origin: 1981
Publisher: Haworth Publishing Company, 28 East 22nd Street, New York, New York 10010. Tel: 212 228 2800
Editor: Robert Hess, Riverwood Community Mental Health Center, 2681 Morton Avenue, St. Joseph, Missouri 49085
Subscription Rate: $32 one-year Individual, $48 one-year Institution, $65 one-year Library
Circulation/Frequency:

Unavailable/Quarterly
Pages per Issue: Variable
Author Payment: None
Photo Policy: Photos Not Accepted
Writer's Guidelines: Contact Editor
Scope of Journal: A first—and in many cases, primary—source of information for mental health and human services developments. Each issue of this theme-oriented journal focuses on a critical problem area providing intensive coverage of that area of prevention.

Preventive Medicine
Year of Origin: 1972
Publisher: Academic Press, c/o American Health Foundation, 320 East 43rd Street, New York, New York 10017. Tel: 212 953 1900
Editor: Ernst L. Wynder, MD
Subscription Rate: $98 Institutional USA, $113 Institutional Foreign, $49 Personal USA; $26.50 Student, $61 Personal Foreign; $35.50 Student
Circulation/Frequency: 1,200/Bi-monthly
Pages per Issue: 125
Author Payment: Complimentary Copy
Photo Policy: Black and White Glossies Accepted
Scope of Journal: This journal provides an international medium for the publication of original manuscripts dealing with applied research into all aspects of prevention. While the emphasis is on heart disease, cancer, and stroke, manuscripts dealing with all leading causes of death, particularly those deemed preventable are eligible for inclusion in the periodical. The editor invites papers from investigators in any scientific discipline whose findings apply to the reduction of disease and death.

Primary Care
Year of Origin: 1974
Publisher: W. B. Saunders, West
Washington Square, Philadelphia,
Pennsylvania 19105. Tel: 215 574
4700
Editor: Guest Editor For Each Issue
Subscription Rate: $32 one-year
Circulation/Frequency:
Unavailable/Quarterly
Pages per Issue: about 250
Author Payment: None
Photo Policy: Black and White Glossies
Scope of Journal: Hard cover periodical. Each issue is focused on a specific topic and contains 10 to 15 state-of-the-art reviews on current clinical practice by leading specialists in the field. Unsolicited articles are not accepted. The "guest editor" of each issue invites papers on areas of current interest.

Primary Care: Clinics In Office Practice
Year of Origin: 1974
Publisher: W. B. Saunders Company,
West Washington Square, Philadelphia, Pennsylvania 19105. Tel: 215
574 4822
Editor: Kay Dowgun
Subscription Rate: $32 one-year
Circulation/Frequency: 10,000/Quarterly
Pages per Issue: 224
Author Payment: None
Photo Policy: Black and White Glossies
Writer's Guidelines: No unsolicited articles, Contact Editor
Scope of Journal: This journal does not have as much research orientation as clinical and practical reviews related to diagnosis and management in the area of primary care.

The Proceedings of the Nutrition Society
Year of Origin: 1941
Publisher: Cambridge University
Press, 32 East 57th Street, New York,
New York 10022. Tel: 212 688 8885
Editor: R. H. Smith
Subscription Rate: $125 one-year
Circulation/Frequency: 2,558/3 yearly
Pages per Issue: 120–170
Author Payment: None
Photo Policy: Photos Not Accepted
Scope of Journal: This journal contains complete records of invited papers read at the Symposium of the Nutrition Society and abstracts of communications which were summaries of papers read by members at the Society's scientific meetings. Occasionally reports or comments of special interest in the field of nutrition are printed.

Prostaglandins Bibliography
Year of Origin: 1960
Publisher: Medical Documentation
Service, 19 South 22nd Street,
Philadelphia, Pennsylvania 19103.
Tel: 1 215 563 1238
Editor: Alberta D. Berton, Dr. James
Powell
Subscription Rate: Yearly Variance
Circulation/Frequency: 1,000/Annually
Pages per Issue: 800–1,000
Author Payment: None
Photo Policy: Photos Not Accepted
Writer's Guidelines: Not Applicable
Scope of Journal: This bibliography uses abbreviations in accordance with the Word-Abbreviation List of the American National Standards Institute. Articles are listed in alphabetical order by author. The primary sort is made by the first three authors, secondary sort is by year of article.

Psychiatric Annals
Year of Origin: 1971
Publisher: Charles B. Slack, Inc.,
6900 Grove Road, Thorofare, New
Jersey 08086. Tel: 609 848 1000
Editor: Howard P. Rome, MD, Francis J. Braceland, MD (Editorial Directors)
Subscription Rate: $30 one-year
Circulation/Frequency:
28,000/Monthly
Pages per Issue: 60–85
Author Payment: None
Photo Policy: Photos Not Accepted
Writer's Guidelines: Contact Editor
Scope of Journal: This journal features articles on new insights and new developments that will affect the practice of psychiatry in the USA. It aims to provide physicians with new information on the diagnosis and management of psychological and psychiatric disorders. The Editorial Directors welcome unsolicited manuscripts that will be useful to the practicing psychiatrist.

Psychiatric Clinics of North America
Year of Origin: 1978
Publisher: W. B. Saunders, West Washington Square, Philadelphia, Pennsylvania 19105. Tel: 215 574 4700
Editor: Guest Editor For Each Issue
Subscription Rate: $39 one-year
Circulation/Frequency: Unavailable/3 yearly
Pages per Issue: about 250
Author Payment: None
Photo Policy: Black and White Glossies
Scope of Journal: Hard cover periodicals. Each issue is focused on a specific topic and contains 10 to 15 state-of-the-art reviews on current clinical practice by leading specialists in the field. Unsolicited articles are not accepted. The "guest editor" of

each issue invites papers on areas of current interest.

Psychiatric Quarterly: A Publication of the New York School of Psychiatry
Year of Origin: 1932
Publisher: Human Science Press, 72 Fifth Avenue, New York, New York 10011. Tel: 212 243 6000
Editor: Raul Vispo
Subscription Rate: $62 Institution, $28 Individual
Circulation/Frequency: 1,100/Quarterly
Pages per Issue: 80 average
Author Payment: None
Photo Policy: Black and White Glossies
Writer's Guidelines: No Specific Guidelines; Use Format Within Journal
Scope of Journal: This journal has two major objectives: to be an independent voice, openly speaking its mind in the field of mental illness care and to assist mental health professionals, particularly those in the policymaking areas in keeping up with pertinent scientific and delivery system data. In addition to highly selective articles, each issue will feature one or more reviews of the social, clinical, administrative, legal, political, and ethnical aspects of mental illness.

Psychiatry: Journal for the Study of Interpersonal Processes
Year of Origin: 1938
Publisher: The William Alanson White Psychiatric Foundation, 1610 New Hampshire Avenue NW, Washington, D. C. 20009. Tel: 202 667 3008
Editor: Donald L. Burnham, M.D.
Subscription Rate: $30 Institution, $20 Individual (Add $4 For Foreign)

Circulation/Frequency: 2,500/Quarterly
Pages per Issue: 100
Author Payment: None
Photo Policy: Photos Not Accepted
Writer's Guidelines: Upon Request From Publisher
Scope of Journal: This journal seeks to provide a medium for effective communication between psychiatry, the social sciences, and all other branches of the study of man and his individual and collective problems in living. The journal attempts to be broadly communicative without sacrificing technical quality. It is designed to present accounts of clinical and field observations, reports of original research, surveys and critiques of scientific literature, and studies concerning methodology, epistemology, and philosophy.

Psychoanalytic Review
Year of Origin: 1913
Publisher: Human Science Press, 72 Fifth Avenue, New York, New York 10011. Tel: 212 243 6000
Editor: Leila Lerner
Subscription Rate: $58 Institution, $26 Individual
Circulation/Frequency: 2,900/Quarterly
Pages per Issue: 160 average
Author Payment: None
Photo Policy: Black and White Glossies
Writer's Guidelines: No Specific Guidelines; Use Format Within Journal
Scope of Journal: This is the oldest English language journal of psychoanalysis and has become a forum for distinguished clinicians representing all gradations of psychoanalytic opinion.

Psychological Abstracts
Year of Origin: 1927
Publisher: American Psychological Association, 1200 17th Street NW, Washington, D. C. 20036. Tel: 202 833 7624
Editor: Lois Granick
Subscription Rate: $450 one-year (USA), $480 one-year (Foreign)
Circulation/Frequency: 5,000/Monthly
Pages per Issue: 280–300
Author Payment: None
Photo Policy: Photos Not Accepted
Writer's Guidelines: Not Applicable
Scope of Journal: Publishes nonevaluative summaries of the world's literature in psychology and related disciplines. Covers over 1,000 journals, technical reports, monographs, and other documents. Each monthly issue includes approximately 2,300 entries plus subject and author indexes. Twice a year, a Volume Index is published to provide an expanded subject Index and an integrated Author Index.

Psychological Bulletin
Year of Origin: 1904
Publisher: American Psychological Association, 1200 17th Avenue, NW, Washington, D. C. 20036. Tel: 202 833 7686
Editor: David Zeaman
Subscription Rate: $25 one year member, $60 one year nonmember
Circulation/Frequency: 9,800/Bimonthly
Pages per Issue: 19–20
Author Payment: None
Photo Policy: Black and White Glossies
Scope of Journal: Publishes evaluative and integrative reviews and interpretations of substantive and methodological issues in scientific psychology.

Psychological Medicine
Year of Origin: 1970
Publisher: Cambridge University Press, 32 East 57th Street, New York, New York 10022. Tel: 212 688 8885
Editor: Prof. Michael Shepherd
Subscription Rate: $89 one-year Individual, $175.50 one-year Institution
Circulation/Frequency: 1,387/Quarterly
Pages per Issue: 232
Author Payment: None
Photo Policy: Unmounted Black and White Glossies
Scope of Journal: This journal publishes original research in clinical, experimental and psychosocial psychiatry and the basic sciences related to it. In addition to original articles and case reports, the journal publishes editorial and commissioned articles from time to time.

The Psychological Record
Year of Origin: 1937
Publisher: Kenyon College, Gambier, Ohio 43022. 614 427 2244, ext 2377
Editor: Charles E. Rice
Subscription Rate: $32 Institution, $15 Individual, $10 Student
Circulation/Frequency: 1,700/Quarterly
Pages per Issue: 150
Author Payment: Yearly Subscription
Photo Policy: Black and White Glossies (figures)
Scope of Journal: This journal publishes theoretical and experimental articles and commentary on current developments in psychology. Papers that develop new methods are favored; contains book reviews.

Psychological Review
Year of Origin: 1894
Publisher: American Psychological Association, 1200 17th Avenue NW, Washington, D.C. 20036, Tel: 202 833 7686
Editor: Martin L. Hoffman
Subscription Rate: $12 one year member, $26 one year nonmember
Circulation/Frequency: 7,300/Bimonthly
Pages per Issue: 20–21
Author Payment: None
Photo Policy: Black and White Glossies
Writer's Guidelines: Contact Editor
Scope of Journal: Publishes articles that make theoretical contributions to any area of scientific psychology. Preference is given to papers which advance theory rather than review it and to statements which are specifically theoretical rather than programmatic.

Psychological Reports
Year of Origin: 1955
Publisher: R. B Ammons, Box 9229, Missoula, Montana 59807. Tel. 406 243 4902
Editor: R. B. Ammons, C. H. Ammons
Subscription Rate: $132.20 one-year
Circulation/Frequency: International/Bi-monthly
Pages per Issue: 100–115
Author Payment: Author pays $27.50 per page, 50/200 reprints free/by pages
Photo Policy: Black and White Glossies 4½ × 6". Original Drawings
Scope of Journal: The purpose of this journal is to encourage scientific originality and creativity in the field of general psychology, for the person who is first a psychologist, then a specialist. It carries experimental, theoretical, and speculative articles; comments; special reviews; and a listing of new books and other material received. Controversial material of scientific merit is welcomed.

Psychology in the Schools
Year of Origin: 1964
Publisher: Clinical Psychology Publishing Co., Inc., 4 Conant Square, Brandon, Vermont 05733. Tel: 802 247 6871
Editor: G. B. Fuller, Dept. of Psychology, Central Michigan University, Mt. Pleasant, Michigan 48858
Subscription Rate: $50 Institution, $25 Individual
Circulation/Frequency: 2,200/Quarterly
Pages per Issue: 150
Author Payment: None
Photo Policy: Photos Not Accepted
Writer's Guidelines: American Psychological Association Style Manual
Scope of Journal: Publishes recent research in educational psychology, theoretical articles, and book reviews.

Psychology of Women Quarterly
Year of Origin: 1975
Publisher: Human Science Press, 72 Fifth Avenue, New York, New York 10011. Tel: 212 243 6000
Editor: Nancy Henley
Subscription Rate: $54 Institution, $25 Individual
Circulation/Frequency: 3,738/Quarterly
Pages per Issue: 100 average
Author Payment: None
Photo Policy: Black and White Glossies
Writer's Guidelines: No Specific Guidelines; Use Format Within Journal
Scope of Journal: This quarterly publishes the most current and important findings now occurring in the area of female psychology. Among the subjects covered are personality development, psychodynamics, socialization, psychobiology, female sexuality, psychopathology, psychotherapy, child development, and child-rearing, creativity, career development, and leadership training.

Psychosocial Rehabilitation Journal
Year of Origin: 1977
Publisher: Boston University, Center for Rehabilitation Research and Training in Mental Health, 1019 Commonwealth Avenue, Boston, Massachusetts 02215. Tel: 617 353 3549
Editor: LeRoy Spaniol
Subscription Rate: $18 USA Individual, $26 USA Institution, $10 USA Student, $26 Foreign Individual, $32 Foreign Institution, $26 Foreign Student
Circulation/Frequency: 1,200/Quarterly
Pages per Issue: 40–45
Author Payment: 60% contributed
Photo Policy: Photos Not Accepted
Scope of Journal: The purpose of this journal is to encourage the communication of information relevant to the rehabilitation of persons with psychiatric disabilities, with the goal of improving the quality of services designed to help in the community adjustment of persons who are psychiatrically disabled. Publishes information on innovative service programs, new research efforts, and current thinking with respect to issues of policy and administration.

Psychosomatic Medicine
Publisher: American Psychosomatic Society, Elsevier North-Holland, Inc., 52 Vanderbilt Avenue, New York, New York, 10017. Tel: 516 379 0191
Editor: Donald Oken, 265 Nassau Road, Roosevelt, New York 11575
Subscription Rate: $49 one-year Individual, $98 one-year Institution, $16 one-year Member
Circulation/Frequency: 2,790/Bimonthly
Pages per Issue: 83 average

Author Payment: None
Photo Policy: Photos Not Accepted
Scope of Journal: This journal includes articles on the psychological, psychiatric, and medical aspects of psychosomatic disease.

Psychosomatics
Year of Origin: 1960
Publisher: Ronald E. March, 500 West Putnam Avenue, Greenwich, Connecticut 06830.
Editor: Leo Christofar
Subscription Rate: $20 USA, $22 Foreign
Circulation/Frequency: 32, 942/ Monthly
Pages Per Issue: 104–120
Author Payment: None
Photo Policy: Photos Not Accepted
Scope of Journal: Timely, practical, peer-reviewed articles on mind-body interactions and the role of psychiatry in the daily practice of comprehensive medicine.

PsycSCAN: Applied Psychology
Year of Origin: 1981
Publisher: American Psychological Association, 1200 17th Street NW, Washington D. C. 20036. Tel: 202 833 7624
Editor: Lois Granick
Subscription Rate: $12 one-year (USA), $15 one-year (Foreign)
Circulation/Frequency: 3,000/Quarterly
Pages per Issue: 60–70
Author Payment: None
Photo Policy: Photos Not Accepted
Writer's Guidelines: Contact Publisher
Scope of Journal: This publication includes abstracts previously published in *Psychological Abstracts* from approximately 55 subscriber-selected journals in the area of applied psychology.

PsycSCAN: Clinical Psychology
Year of Origin: 1980
Publisher: American Psychological Association, 1200 17th Street NW, Washington, D. C. 20036. Tel: 202 833 7624
Editor: Lois Granick
Subscription Rate: $12 one-year (USA), $15 one-year (Foreign)
Circulation/Frequency: 7,500/Quarterly
Pages per Issue: 50–60
Author Payment: None
Photo Policy: Photos Not Accepted
Writer's Guidelines: Contact Publisher
Scope of Journal: This publication includes abstracts previously published in *Psychological Abstracts* from approximately 20 subscriber selected journals in the area of clinical psychology.

PsycSCAN: Developmental Psychology
Year of Origin: 1980
Publisher: American Psychological Association, 1200 17th Street NW, Washington, D. C. 20036. Tel: 202 833 7624
Editor: Lois Granick
Subscription Rate: $12 one-year (USA), $15 one-year (Foreign)
Circulation/Frequency: 3,200/Quarterly
Pages per Issue: about 60
Author Payment: None
Photo Policy: Photos Not Accepted
Writer's Guidelines: Contact Publisher
Scope of Journal: This publication includes abstracts previously published in *Psychological Abstracts* from approximately 30 subscriber-selected journals in the area of developmental psychology.

PsycSCAN: Learning Disabilities, Mental Retardation
Year of Origin: 1982
Publisher: American Psychological Association, 1200 17th Street NW, Washington, D. C. 20036. Tel: 202 833 7624
Editor: Lois Granick
Subscription Rate: $12 one-year (USA), $15 one-year (Foreign)
Circulation/Frequency: Quarterly
Pages per Issue: about 60
Author Payment: None
Photo Policy: Photos Not Accepted
Writer's Guidelines: Contact Publisher
Scope of Journal: This publication includes abstracts previously published in *Psychological Abstracts* using for selection criteria a core group of index terms in the areas of learning disabilities, communication disorders, and mental retardation.

Public Health Reports
Year of Origin: 1878
Publisher: U. S. Public Health Service, 814 Reporters Bldg., Washington, D. C. 20201. Tel: 202 426 5146
Editor: Marian Priest Tebben
Subscription Rate: $18 one-year
Circulation/Frequency: 12,000/Bimonthly
Pages per Issue: 96
Author Payment: None
Photo Policy: Black and White Glossies
Scope of Journal: Publishes scientific and research articles on public health and community medicine issues.

Radiologic Clinics of North America
Year of Origin: 1963
Publisher: W. B. Saunders, West Washington Square, Philadelphia, Pennsylvania 19105. Tel: 215 574 4700
Editor: Guest Editor For Each Issue
Subscription Rate: $40 one-year

Circulation/Frequency: Unavailable/Bi-monthly
Pages per Issue: about 250
Author Payment: None
Photo Policy: Black and White Glossies
Scope of Journal: Hard cover periodical. Each issue is focused on a specific topic and contains 10 to 15 state-of-the-art reviews on current clinical practice by leading specialists in the field. Unsolicited articles are not accepted. The "guest editor" of each issue invites papers on areas of current interest.

Radiologic Technology
Year of Origin: 1970
Publisher: Charles B. Slack, Inc., 6900 Grove Road, Thorofare, New Jersey 08086. Tel: 609 848 1000
Editor: Pamela Wight
Subscription Rate: $25 one-year
Circulation/Frequency: 20,200/Bi-monthly
Pages per issue: 80
Author Payment: None
Photo Policy: Black and White Glossies 5 × 7
Scope of Journal: The purpose of this journal is to provide current information by well-informed professionals in the field of Radiologic Technology in an interesting, readable fashion with attention to relevance in the state of the art.

Regional Anesthesia
Year of Origin: 1940
Publisher: J. B. Lippincott Company, East Washington Square, Philadelphia, Pennsylvania 19105. Tel: 215 574 4216
Editor: Harold Carron, MD, Box 238, Medical Center, University of Virginia, Charlottesville, Virginia 22908
Subscription Rate: $20 one-year USA,

$50 one-year Foreign
Circulation/Frequency:
29,179/Monthly
Pages per Issue: about 50
Author Payment: None
Photo Policy: Black and White Glossies up to 5 × 7
Scope of Journal: This journal is designed for publication of research papers and other articles of highest quality relevant to the practitioner concerned with local anesthetics and regional anesthesia.

Retina
Year of Origin: 1981
Publisher: J. B. Lippincott Company, East Washington Square, Philadelphia, Pennsylvania 19105. Tel: 215 574 4216
Editor: A. J. Brucker, M. D., Box 67, Gladwyne, Pennsylvania, 19035
Subscription Rate: $45 one-year USA, $55 one-year Foreign
Circulation/Frequency: 1,614/Quarterly
Pages per Issue: 50–70
Author Payment: None
Photo Policy: Black and White Glossies up to 8 × 10
Scope of Journal: This is a journal of retinal and vitreous diseases and publishes original and special articles concerning disorders of the retina and vitreous. Manuscripts will be reviewed by two or more reviewers.

Review of Educational Research
Year of Origin: 1931
Publisher: American Educational Research Association, 1230 17th Street NW, Washington, D. C. 20036. Tel: 202 223 9485
Editor: Dr. Naftaly Glasman
Subscription Rate: $16 one-year Individual, $21 one-year Institution, $12 one-year Member
Circulation/Frequency: 15,000/Quarterly
Pages per Issue: 160
Author Payment: None
Photo Policy: Camera Ready Accepted
Scope of Journal: Publishes critical, integrative reviews of research literature bearing on education. It includes reviews and interpretations of substantive and methodological issues relevant to education from any discipline such as reviews of research in biology, psychology, evaluation, humanities, political science, sociology and other health-related fields provided that the reviews bear on educational issues.

Scientific American
Year of Origin: about 1960
Publisher: Gerard Piel, 415 Madison Avenue, New York, New York 10017. Tel: 212 754 0550
Editor: Dennis Flanagan
Subscription Rate: $21 one year USA, $27 one year Foreign
Circulation/Frequency: 721, 339/Monthly
Pages per Issue: 192 Domestic, 152 International
Author Payment: Negotiated
Photo Policy: Negotiated
Writer's Guidelines: None
Scope of Journal: Publishes articles across the full range of science, technology and medicine for the reader strongly interested in progress in those fields. Most of the articles in the magazine are written by those describing their own work.

Sex Roles: A Journal of Research
Year of Origin: 1975
Publisher: Plenum Publishing Company, 233 Spring Street, New York, New York 10013. Tel: 212 620 8466
Editor: Phyllis A. Katz
Subscription Rate: $115 one-year

USA, $133 one-year Foreign
Circulation/Frequency:
Unavailable/Monthly
Pages per Issue: 110
Author Payment: None
Photo Policy: large black and white glossies
Scope of Journal: Publishes an array of articles, materials, etc. pertinent to students and professionals in sex education, sex therapy and social sciences; contains book reviews.

Sexually Transmitted Diseases
Year of Origin: 1974
Publisher: J. B. Lippincott Company, East Washington Square, Philadelphia, Pennsylvania 19105. Tel: 215 574 4216
Editor: William M. McCormack, MD
Subscription Rate: $37 one-year USA, $41 one-year Foreign
Circulation/Frequency: 2,514/Quarterly
Pages per Issue: 50–70
Author Payment: None
Photo Policy: Photos Not Accepted
Scope of Journal: This journal welcomes papers on clinical, laboratory, epidemiologic, sociologic, and historical topics pertinent to sexually transmitted diseases and related fields. The following types are suitable: original articles, notes, reviews, editorials, and letters.

Small Group Behavior
Year of Origin: 1971
Publisher: Sage Publications, Inc., 275 South Beverly Drive, Beverly Hills, California 90213. Tel: 213 274 8003
Editor: Fred Massarik, University of California, Los Angeles
Subscription Rate: $46 one-year Institution, $22 one-year Individual, $91 two-year Institution, $43 two-year Individual, $136 three-year Institution, $64 three-year Individual

Circulation/Frequency: 900/Quarterly
Pages per Issue: 120–130
Author Payment: Complimentary Copies of Journal
Photo Policy: Photos Not Accepted
Writer's Guidelines: Contact Publisher
Scope of Journal: An international and interdisciplinary journal presenting the newest theory and research on all types of small groups. The journal reports on qualitative and quantitative measures and methods, and looks at groups in both natural and experimental settings. Brief reports on works-in-progress, new ideas, book reviews and news of professional events are welcome.

Smoking and Health
Year of Origin: 1968
Publisher: Department of Health and Human Services, 5600 Fishers Lane (Park 158), Public Health Service, Rockville, Maryland 20857. Tel: 301 443 1690
Editor: Donald R. Shopland
Subscription Rate: free
Circulation/Frequency: 5,200/six yearly
Pages per Issue: 75
Author Payment: None
Photo Policy: Photos Not Accepted
Writer's Guidelines: Contact Editor
Scope of Journal: Publishes a variety of articles, materials, reports important to researchers on the topic of the health hazards of smoking; includes citations and abstracts.

Smoking and Health Bibliography
Year of Origin: 1968
Publisher: Department of Health and Human Services, 5600 Fishers Lane (Park 158), Public Health Service, Rockville, Maryland 20857. Tel: 301 443 1690
Editor: Donald R. Shopland
Subscription Rate: free

Circulation/Frequency: 5,000/Annually
Pages per Issue: 530
Author Payment: Not Applicable
Photo Policy: Not Applicable
Writer's Guidelines: Not Applicable
Scope of Journal: A cumulative subject and author index based on the *Smoking and Health Builletin.*

Social Casework: The Journal of Contemporary Social Work
Year of Origin: 1920
Publisher: Family Service Association of America, 44 East 23rd Street, New York, New York 10010. Tel: 212 674 6100
Editor: Robert A. Eilfers
Subscription Rate: $22 one-year Individual, $33 one-year Institution
Circulation/Frequency: 14,000/Monthly, Except July/August
Pages per Issue: 64
Author Payment: None
Photo Policy: Photos Not Accepted
Scope of Journal: A refereed journal directed primarily to the interests of social work practitioners and educators. Preference is given to articles that illuminate a facet of social work theory or practice and that report professional concerns of social workers.

Social Cognition
Year of Origin: March 1982
Publisher: The Guilford Press, 200 Park Avenue South, New York, New York 10003
Editor: David J. Schneider, Division of Social Sciences, University of Texas, San Antonio, Texas. Tel: 1 512 691 4375
Subscription Rate: $45 one-year USA, $55 one-year Foreign
Circulation/Frequency: abt 1,000/Quarterly
Pages per Issue: 100
Author Payment: None

Photo Policy: Camera-ready
Scope of Journal: This journal publishes reports of empirical research, conceptual analyses, and critical reviews of the role of cognitive processes in the study of personality, development, and social behavior. It emphasizes three broad concerns: the ways people perceive, code, manipulate and remember socially relevant stimuli; the effects of social, cultural, and affective factors on the processing of information; the behavioral and interpersonal consequences of cognitive processes.

Social Indicators Research
Year of Origin: 1974
Publisher: D. Reidel Publishing Company, Box 17, 3300 AA Dordrecht, Holland
Editor: A.C. Michalos
Subscription Rate: $20 USA Individuals, $67.50 USA Institutions
Circulation/Frequency: 900/8 yearly
Pages per Issue: 110
Author Payment: None
Photo Policy: Photos Not Accepted
Scope of Journal: This journal has emerged as the leading publication dealing with problems relating to the measurement of all aspects of the quality of life. The studies include: empirical, philosophical, and methodological and take in the whole spectrum of society i.e. individual, public and private organizations, and municipal, county, regional, national, and international systems.

Social Psychology Quarterly, Previously: Sociometry, Social Psychology
Year of Origin: 1937
Publisher: American Sociological Association, 1722 North Street NW, Washington, D. C. 20036. Tel: 202 833 3410
Editor: George W. Bohrnstedt

Subscription Rate: $19 Institution, $14 Individual, $8 Members
Circulation/Frequency: 5,000/Quarterly
Pages per Issue: 64–70
Author Payment: $10 Processing Fee Required
Photo Policy: Photos Not Accepted
Scope of Journal: This journal publishes papers pertaining to the processes and products of social interaction. This includes the study of the primary relations of individuals to one another, or to groups, or institutions, and also the study of intra-individual processes in so far as they substantially influence, or are influenced by, social forces.

Social Research
Year of Origin: 1934
Publisher: New School for Social Research, 65 Fifth Avenue, New York, New York 10003. Tel: 212 741 5776
Editor: Dr. Arien Mack
Subscription Rate: $35 Institution, $20 Individual
Circulation/Frequency: 3,600/Quarterly
Pages per Issue: 200
Author Payment: None
Photo Policy: Photos Not Accepted
Scope of Journal: This journal emphasized interdisciplinary treatment of issues in social sciences and seeks to maintain the humanistic tradition by integration with the approaches of philosophy and history.

Social Science and Medicine: An International Journal
Year of Origin: 1966
Publisher: The Pergamon Press, Maxwell House, Fairview Park, Elmsford, New York, 10523. Tel: 914 592 7700
Editor: Dr. Peter J. M. McEwan
Subscription Rate: $450 one-year
Circulation/Frequency: 2,000/24 yearly

Pages per Issue: 2,400
Author Payment: None
Photo Policy: Photos Not Accepted
Scope of Journal: This journal was established to aid the dissemination of important research and theoretical work in all areas of common interest to the socio-behavioural sciences and medicine, including psychiatry and epidemiology; also, to exchange ideas and information throughout the world among those engaged in different disciplines who are focusing their attention on aspects of the inter-relationships between the various branches of medicine and the social sciences.

Social Work in Health Care
Year of Origin: 1975
Publisher: Haworth Publishing Company, 28 East 22nd Street, New York, New York 10010. Tel: 212 228 2800
Editor: Sylvia S. Clarke, Special Consultant, Department of Social Work Services, Mount Sinair Hospital, 1 Gustave C. Levy Place, New York, New York 10029
Subscription Rate: $32 one-year Individual, $48 one-year Institution, $60 one-year Library
Circulation/Frequency: 3,400/Quarterly
Pages per Issue: Variable
Author Payment: None
Photo Policy: Photos Not Accepted
Writer's Guidelines: Contact Editor
Scope of Journal: This is an interdisciplinary journal devoted to theory, practice, and administration in a wide variety of health care settings. Covers issues in patient services and family counseling.

Sociological Quarterly
Year of Origin: 1939
Publisher: Department of Sociology, Southern Illinois University, Carbondale, Illinois 62901. Tel: 618 453 2494
Editor: Thomas G. Eynon
Subscription Rate: $12 one-year
Circulation/Frequency: 2,500/Quarterly
Pages per Issue: 160
Author Payment: None
Photo Policy: Photos Not Accepted
Writer's Guidelines: Contact Publisher
Scope of Journal: Any article in any field of sociological interest.

Southern Medical Journal
Year of Origin: 1906
Publisher: Southern Medical Association, 2601 Highland Avenue, Box 2446, Birmingham, Alabama 35201. Tel: 205 323 4400
Editor: Dr. John B. Thomison
Subscription Rate: $35 one-year
Circulation/Frequency: 25,000/Monthly
Pages per Issue: 120
Author Payment: None
Photo Policy: Black and White Glossies
Writer's Guidelines: Included in each journal
Scope of Journal: The purpose of this journal is to foster and develop scientific medicine devoted solely to continuing education. The journal publishes annually more than 450 original clinical articles directed to the practicing physician and surgeon.

Special Care in Dentistry
Year of Origin: 1981
Publisher: American Dental Association, 211 East Chicago Avenue, Chicago, Illinois 60611. Tel: 312 440 2782
Editor: Sidney Epstein, DDS, William Posnick, DDS, Raymond Zambito, DDS
Subscription Rate: $12 one-year USA, $16 one-year Foreign
Circulation/Frequency: 3,000/Bimonthly
Pages per Issue: about 50
Author Payment: None
Photo Policy: Photos Not Accepted
Scope of Journal: The mission of *Special Care* is to enhance communication among those participating in the initiative to elevate the quality of life of patients with needs requiring special attention. The concept will include anyone requiring special attention because of any barrier to dental care, whether it be physical, emotional, financial, or geographic.

Spine
Year of Origin: 1976
Publisher: J. B. Lippincott Company, East Washington Square, Philadelphia, Pennsylvania 19105. Tel: 215 574 4200
Editor: Henry La Rocca, M.D., 4938 Prytania Street, New Orleans, Louisiana 70115
Subscription Rate: $68 one-year USA, $74 one-year Foreign
Circulation/Frequency: 6,152/8 yearly
Pages per Issue: 70–90
Author Payment: None
Photo Policy: Black and White Glossies
Scope of Journal: Original papers are considered for publication with the understanding that they are contributed solely to SPINE. The journal does not publish articles reporting material that has been reported at length elsewhere.

Stroke—A Journal of Cerebral Circulation
Year of Origin: 1970
Publisher: American Heart Association, 7320 Greenville Avenue, Dallas, Texas 75231. Tel: 214 750 5300
Editor: H. J. M. Barnett, MD
Subscription Rate: $40 one-year USA, $55 one-year Foreign
Circulation/Frequency: 5,000/6 yearly
Pages per Issue: Variable
Author Payment: None
Photo Policy: Black and White or Color, Color Cost paid by author
Scope of Journal: A scientific journal concerned with stroke. It is of interest to the practicing physician—especially the internist, cardiologist and neurologist—as well as a teacher, a clinical investigator, laboratory scientist and student. Articles include clinical conferences and deal with prevention, diagnosis, treatment and rehabilitation.

Studies in Family Planning
Year of Origin: 1963
Publisher: The Population Council, One Dag Hammarskjold Plaza, New York, New York 10017. Tel: 212 644 1300
Editor: Valeda Slade
Subscription Rate: Free to professionals in the population field; Back Issues: 75¢/copy, Special Issues: $2.50/copy
Circulation/Frequency: 8,000/Monthly
Pages per Issue: 32–48
Author Payment: None
Photo Policy: Photos Not Accepted
Writer's Guidelines: Contact Publisher
Scope of Journal: This publication is an international journal devoted to articles and commentary on all aspects of fertility control and family planning with particular emphasis on activities in the developing countries. Areas of interest include advances in contraceptive technology, efficacy, and safety; the interface of women's roles and status with family planning; consumer's perspective; and the health, social, political, and economic impacts of fertility regulation policies and programs.

Suicide and Life-Threatening Behavior
Year of Origin: 1969
Publisher: Human Science Press, 72 Fifth Avenue, New York, New York 10011. 212 243 6000
Editor: Ronald W. Maris
Subscription Rate: $70 Institution; $29 Individual
Circulation/Frequency: 1,525/Quarterly
Pages per Issue: 80 average
Author Payment: None
Photo Policy: Black and White Glossies
Writer's Guidelines: No Specific Guidelines; Use Format Within Journal
Scope of Journal: This journal is devoted to emergent approaches in theory and practice relating to self-destructive, other-destructive and life threatening behaviors. It is multidisciplinary and concerned with a variety of topics, such as: suicide prevention, death, accidents, subintentioned destruction, partial death-threats to life's length, and breadth from within and without.

Surgery
Year of Origin: 1937
Publisher: The C. V. Mosby Company, 11830 Westline Industrial Drive, St. Louis, Missouri 63141. Tel: 314 872 8370
Editor: Walter F. Ballinger, MD, Washington University School of Medicine, George D. Zuidema, MD, Johns Hopkins Hospital

Subscription Rate: $56.50 one-year Institution USA, $70.00 International, $35.50 one-year Individual USA, $49.00 International, $28.40 one-year Student USA, $41.90 International
Circulation/Frequency: 11,872/Monthly
Pages per Issue: 135
Author Payment: None
Photo Policy: Black and White Glossies
Scope of Journal: This is the official journal for Society of University Surgeons, Society for Vascular Surgery, Central Surgical Association. Articles submitted for publication should be original communications related to this title and submitted exclusively to *Surgery*.

Surgical Clinics of North America
Year of Origin: 1912
Publisher: W. B. Saunders, West Washington Square, Philadelphia, Pennsylvania 19105. Tel: 215 574 4700
Editor: Guest Editor for Each Issue
Subscription Rate: $36 one-year
Circulation/Frequency: Unavailable/Bi-monthly
Pages per Issue: about 250
Author Payment: None
Photo Policy: Black and White Glossies
Scope of Journal: Hard cover periodical. Each issue is focused on a specific topic and contains 10 to 15 state-of-the-art reviews on current clinical practice by leading specialists in the field. Unsolicited articles are not accepted. The "guest editor" of each issue invites papers on areas of current interest.

Texas Heart Institute Journal
Previously: Cardiovascular Diseases, Bulletin of THI
Year of Origin: 1974

Publisher: Texas Heart Institute, Box 20269, Houston, Texas 77225. Tel: 713 791 3121
Editor: Robert J. Hall, MD
Subscription Rate: $15 one-year
Circulation/Frequency: 24,000/Quarterly
Pages per Issue: 110–130
Author Payment: None
Photo Policy: Black and White Glossies 3 × 5"
Scope of Journal: Publishes only medical, research, perfusion and medically related articles.

Today's Education
Year of Origin: 1921
Publisher: National Education Association, 1201 16th Street NW, Washington D. C. 20036. Tel: 202 833 4000
Editor: Elizabeth E. Yeary
Subscription Rate: Membership Fee Includes Journal
Circulation/Frequency: 1.7 million/Quarterly
Pages per Issue: 80
Author Payment: None
Photo Policy: Author Charge For Photo Inclusion, 8 × 10 B & W $50; Color $150
Writer's Guidelines: Contact Editor
Scope of Journal: Consideration is given to any article concerned with current issues in any level of education.

Topics in Emergency Medicine
Year of Origin: 1979
Publisher: Aspen Systems Corporation, 1600 Research Blvd., Rockville, Maryland 20850. Tel: 301 251 5000
Editor: John R. Marozsan
Subscription Rate: $39 one-year
Circulation/Frequency: 6,600/Quarterly
Pages per Issue: 100
Author Payment: None

Photo Policy: Photos Not Accepted
Writer's Guidelines: Contact Editor
Scope of Journal: Publishes articles
on key issues of Emergency Medicine

Topics in Health Care Financing
Year of Origin: 1974
Publisher: Aspen Systems Corporation, 1600 Research Blvd., Rockville, Maryland 20850. Tel: 301 251 5000
Editor: John R. Marozsan
Subscription Rate: $49.75 one-year
Circulation/Frequency: 4,500/Quarterly
Pages per Issue: 100
Author Payment: None
Photo Policy: Black and White Glossies
Scope of Journal: Articles submitted must pertain to Health Care Financing.

Traffic Safety
Year of Origin: 1957 (formerly Public Safety—1927)
Publisher: National Safety Council, 444 North Michigan Avenue, Chicago, Illinois 60611. Tel: 312 527 4800, ext. 422
Editor: Robert B. Overend
Subscription Rate: $11.15 one year members, $13.95 one year nonmembers
Circulation/Frequency: 15,000/Bimonthly
Pages per Issue: 32
Author Payment: None
Photo Policy: Black and White Glossies
Scope of Journal: This publication is directed toward readers who are professionally connected with highway and traffic safety. They include federal, state, and local highway officials; traffic engineers; driver education teachers; trucking company executives and safety directors; members of university safety centers; insurance peo-

ple; local safety councils; political leaders; police; and judges of traffic courts. All articles touch on subjects of interest to these readers including enforcement of drink driver and speed laws, school programs, trends in accidents, seat belts, safety legislation

Transactional Analysis Journal
Year of Origin: about 1966
Publisher: International Transactional Analysis Association, Inc., 1772 Vallejo Street, San Francisco, California 94123. Tel: 415 885 5992
Editor: John R. McNeel, Ph.D.
Subscription Rate: $20 one year
Circulation/Frequency: 6,600/Quarterly
Pages per Issue: 100
Author Payment: None
Photo Policy: Photos Not Accepted
Scope of Journal: This journal publishes an array of articles, materials and announcements pertinent to individuals interested in and involved with transactional analysis.

Transfusion
Year of Origin: 1961
Publisher: J. B. Lippincott Company, East Washington Square, Philadelphia, Pennsylvania 19105. Tel: 215 574 4216
Editor: Thomas F. Zuck, MD
Subscription Rate: $43 one-year USA, $50 one-year Canada/Foreign
Circulation/Frequency: 12,481/Bi-monthly
Pages per Issue: 60–80
Author Payment: Author must pay $25 review fee
Photo Policy: Black and White Glossies, (colored at author's expense)
Scope of Journal: This journal provides an international forum for the publication in English of communications which advance knowledge re-

lated to transfusion therapy, immunohematology, and transplantation. The scope includes all scientific, technical, and administrative aspects of blood banking. Acceptance of papers is based solely on merit; equal consideration is given to nonmembers of the association.

Urologic Clinics of North America
Year of Origin: 1974
Publisher: W. B. Saunders, West Washington Square, Philadelphia, Pennsylvania 19105. Tel: 215 574 4700
Editor: Guest Editor For Each Issue
Subscription Rate: $39 one-year
Circulation/Frequency: Unavailable/Quarterly
Pages per Issue: about 250
Author Payment: None
Photo Policy: Black and White Glossies
Scope of Journal: Hard cover periodical. Each issue is focused on a specific topic and contains 10 to 15 state-of-the-art reviews on current practice by leading specialists in the field. Unsolicited articles are not accepted. The "guest editor" of each issue invites papers on areas of current interest.

Women and Health
Year of Origin: 1976
Publisher: Haworth Publishing Company, 28 East 22nd Street, New York, New York 10010. Tel: 212 228 2800
Editor: Sharon Golub, 32 Runyon Place, Scarsdale, New York 10583
Subscription Rate: $28 one-year Individual, $48 one-year Institution, $65 one-year Library
Circulation/Frequency: 1,095/Quarterly
Pages per Issue: Variable
Author Payment: None
Photo Policy: Photos Not Accepted

Writer's Guidelines: Contact Editor
Scope of Journal: The only scholarly journal devoted exclusively to the broad range of women's health care.

World Health
Year of Origin: 1958
Publisher: World Health Organization (WHO), 1211 Geneva 27, Switzerland. Tel: Central/Exchange: 91 21 11, Direct: 91
Editor: John H. Bland, Division of Public Information
Subscription Rate: $15/annual USA
Circulation/Frequency: 150,000/10 issues annually, eight languages
Pages per Issue: 32 average
Author Payment: £250 per article
Photo Policy: Accepted
Writer's Guidelines: Avoid Jargon
Scope of Journal: This publication seeks to explain the major public health problems, and the World Health Organization's programs for dealing with these problems in terms understandable to the general public. There is a distinct emphasis on the Third World. Articles are commissioned by the Editor: those submitted "on spec" are only very rarely accepted.

Your Life and Health
Year of Origin: 1884
Publisher: Review and Herald Publishing Association, 6856 Eastern Avenue NW, Washington D. C. 20012. Tel: 202 723 3700
Editor: Thomas A. Davis
Subscription Rate: $17.75 one-year
Circulation/Frequency: 50,000/Monthly
Pages per Issue: 32
Author Payment: Articles: $50—$150
Photo Policy: Black and White, Color
Scope of Journal: General articles having to do with mental, social, and physical health.

Professional Association Index

Alliance for the Advancement of Health
  Education
  Health Education, 54
American Academy of Dental Radiology
  Oral Surgery, Oral Medicine, Oral Pathology,
  100
American Academy of Dermatology
  Journal of the American Academy of Dermatology, 64
American Academy of Oral Pathology
  Oral Surgery, Oral Medicine, Oral Pathology,
  100
American Association for Marriage and
  Family Therapy
  Family Therapy, 53
  Family Therapy News, 53
  Journal of Marital and Family Therapy, 77
American Association of Colleges for
  Teacher Education
  Journal of Teacher Education, 88
American Association of Mental Deficiency
  American Journal of Mental Deficiency, 18
  Mental Retardation, 93
American Association of Orthodontists
  American Journal of Orthodontics, 19
American Association of Pathologists
  American Journal of Pathology, 20
American College Health Association
  Journal of the American College Health Association, 64
American Dental Association
  Dental Abstracts, 47
  Journal of the American Dental Association,
  65
  Special Care in Dentistry, 118
American Dental Hygienists' Association
  Dental Hygiene, 47

American Dietetic Association
  Journal of the American Dietetic Association,
  65
American Educational Research Association
  American Educational Research Journal, 14
  Educational Researcher, 49
  Journal of Educational Statistics, 71
  Review of Educational Research, 114
American Geriatrics Society
  Journal of the American Geriatrics Society, 65
American Heart Association
  Circulation, 38
  Circulation Research, 38
  Hypertension, 58
  Modern Concepts of Cardiovascular Disease,
  94
  Stroke—A Journal of Cerebral Circulation,
  119
American Institute of Nutrition
  Journal of Nutrition, 79
American Institute of Oral Biology
  Oral Surgery, Oral Medicine, Oral Pathology,
  100
American Medical Association
  Journal of the American Medical Association,
  65
American Nurses' Association
  American Journal of Nursing, 19
  Nursing Research, 97
American Orthopaedic Society
  American Journal of Sports Medicine, 23
American Orthopsychiatric Association
  American Journal of Orthopsychiatry, 20
American Physiological Society
  American Journal of Physiology, 20
  Physiological Reviews, 104
  The Physiologist, 105

American Psychiatric Association
  American Journal of Psychiatry, 22
American Psychological Association
  American Psychologist, 23
  Journal of Applied Psychology, 67
  Journal of Consulting and Clinical Psychology, 69
  Journal of Counseling Psychology, 70
  Journal of Personality and Social Psychology, 82
  Psychological Bulletin, 109
  Psychological Review, 110
American Psychosomatic Society
  Psychosomatic Medicine, 111
American Public Health Association
  American Journal of Public Health, 23
  The Nation's Health, 95
American School Health Association
  Journal of School Health, 85
American Society for Artificial Internal Organs
  American Society for Artificial Internal Organs Journal, 25
American Society for Surgery of the Hand, The
  The Journal of Hand Surgery, 74
American Society of Clinical Nutrition
  American Journal of Clinical Nutrition, 15
American Society of Clinical Pathologists
  Laboratory Medicine, 90
American Society of Hematology
  Blood, 32
American Society of Law and Medicine
  Law, Medicine, and Health Care, 90
American Society of Microbiology
  Journal of Bacteriology, 67
American Sociological Association
  Social Psychology Quarterly, 116
American Speech-Language-Hearing Association
  Journal of Speech and Hearing Disorders, 87
  Journal of Speech and Hearing Research, 88
  Language-Speech-and-Hearing Services in Schools, 90
American Thoracic Society
  American Review of Respiratory Disease, 24
Association for Childhood Education International
  Childhood Education, 37

Association for Practitioners in Infection Control
  American Journal of Infection Control, 17
Association for Research in Vision and Ophthalmology
  Investigative Ophthalmology and Visual Science, 63
Association for the Advancement of Psychotherapy
  American Journal of Psychotherapy, 22
Association for Thoracic Surgery
  Journal of Thoracic and Cardiovascular Surgery, 89
Association of Operating Room Nurses
  Association of Operating Room Nurses, 30

British Psychological Society
  British Journal of Medical Psychology, 33

Canadian Hospital Association
  Dimensions in Health Science, 48
Canadian Medical Association
  Canadian Medical Association Journal, 35
Canadian Public Health Association
  Canadian Journal of Public Health, 35
Central Surgical Association
  Surgery, 119

Emergency Department Nurses Association
  Journal of Emergency Nursing, 72

International Association for Enterostomal Therapy
  Journal of Enterostomal Therapy, 72
International Council of Nurses
  International Nursing Review, 62
International Union of Microbiological Societies
  International Journal of Systematic Bacteriology, 62

National Association of Pediatric Nurses, Associates and Practitioners
  Pediatric Nursing, 103
National Council for International Health
  International Health News, 59
National Dairy Council
  Dairy Council Digest, 47
  Nutrition News, 97

National Education Association
   Today's Education, 120
National Environmental Health Association
   Journal of Environmental Health, 72
National Intravenous Therapy Association
   National Intravenous Therapy Association Journal, 94
National Safety Council
   Traffic Safety, 121
Nurses Association of Jamaica
   The Jamaican Nurse, 63
Nurses Association of the American College of Obstetricians and Gynecologists
   Journal of Obstetric, Gynecologic, and Neonatal Nursing, 80

Society for Vascular Surgery
   Surgery, 119
Society of University Surgeons
   Surgery, 119
Southern Medical Association
   Southern Medical Journal, 118

World Health Organization
   World Health, 122

Subject, Title and Key Word Index

Adolescence: *Adolescence,* 12
                        Child and Adolescent Social Work Journal, 36
                        Journal of Youth and Adolescence, 89
Aging: *Activities, Adaptation, and Aging,* 11
                        Clinical Gerontologist, 40
                        International Journal of Aging and Human Development, 60
                        Journal of Gerontological Social Work, 73
                        Journal of Housing for the Elderly, 75
                        Journal of Nutrition for the Elderly, 80
                        Journal of the American Geriatric Society, 65
                        Physical and Occupational Therapy and Geriatrics, 104
Allergy: *Clinical Allergy,* 39
                        Journal of Allergy and Clinical Immunology, 64
Anesthesiology: *Anesthesiology,* 25
                        Regional Anesthesia, 113
Artificial Organs: *American Society for Artificial Organs,* 25

Bacteriology: *International Journal of Systematic Bacteriology,* 62
                        Journal of Applied Bacteriology, 66
                        Journal of Bacteriology, 67
Behavior: *Addictive Behaviors,* 11
                        Advances in Behavior Research and Therapy, 13
                        American Behavioral Scientist, 14
                        Archives of Sexual Behavior, 29
                        Behavioral Counseling and Community Interventions, 30
                        Behavioral Science, 31
                        Behavior Research and Therapy, 31
                        Child and Family Behavior Therapy, 37
                        Imagination, Cognition, and Personality, 58
                        Journal of Applied Behavioral Science, 66
                        Journal of Applied Behavior Analysis, 66
                        Journal of Behavioral Medicine, 67
                        Journal of Behavior Therapy and Experimental Psychiatry, 68
                        Journal of Nonverbal Behavior, 78
                        Journal of Organizational Behavior Management, 82
                        Small Group Behavior, 115

	Social Cognition, 116
	Suicide and Life-Threatening Behavior, 119
Biochemistry:	*Annual Review of Biochemistry,* 26
Bioethics:	*Biofeedback and Self-Regulation, 31*
	Journal of Bioethics, 68
Biology:	*Pavlovian Journal of Biological Science,* 102
	Perspectives in Biology and Medicine, 103
Cancer:	*Breast Cancer Research and Treatment,* 32
	Cancer, 35
	Cancer Mestasis Reviews, 36
	Cancer Research, 36
	Journal of Neuro-Oncology, 78
Child:	*Care, Health and Development,* 37
Child Care:	*Child Care Quarterly,* 37
	Clinical Pediatrics, 41
	Journal of Pediatrics, 82
	Merrill-Palmer Quarterly, 93
	Pediatric Annals, 102
	Pediatric Clinics of North America, 102
	Pediatric Nursing, 103
	Physical and Occupational Therapy in Pediatrics, 104
Circulatory Health:	*American Journal of Cardiology,* 15
	Arteriosclerosis: A Journal of Vascular Biology and Disease, 29
	Blood, 32
	British Journal of Haematology, 33
	Heart and Lung: The Journal of Critical Care, 56
	Hypertension, 58
	Journal of Thoracic and Cardiovascular Surgery, 89
	Modern Concepts of Cardiovascular Disease, 94
	National Intravenous Therapy Association, 94
	Stroke—A Journal of Cerebral Circulation, 119
	Texas Heart Institute Journal, 120
	Transfusion, 122
College Health:	*Journal of the American College Health Association,* 122
Community Health:	*Community Mental Health Journal,* 45
	Family and Community Health, 52
	International Quarterly of Community Health Education, 62
	Journal of Community Health, 69
Counseling:	*Behavior Counseling and Community Interventions,* 30
	Journal of Counseling Psychology, 70
	Patient Education and Counseling, 102
Death:	*Omega: Journal of Death and Dying,* 99
Dental Health:	*Dental Abstracts,* 47
	Dental Clinics of North America, 47
	Dental Hygiene, 47
	Journal of Prosthetic Dentistry, 83

                    Journal of the American Dental Association, 65
                    Special Care in Denistry, 118

Dermatology: *British Journal of Dermatology,* 33
                    Journal of the American Academy of Dermatology, 64

Dietetics: *Journal of the American Dietetic Association,* 65

Disease: *American Journal of Digestive Diseases,* 16
                    American Journal of Diseases of Children, 17
                    American Journal of Infection Control, 17
                    American Review of Respiratory Disease, 24
                    Arteriosclerosis: A Journal of Vascular Biology and Disease, 29
                    Breast Cancer Research and Treatment, 32
                    Cancer, 35
                    Clinics in Rheumatic Diseases, 45
                    Diseases of the Colon and Rectum, 48
                    Journal of Chronic Diseases, 68
                    Journal of Infectious Diseases, 76
                    Modern Concepts of Cardiovascular Disease, 94
                    Sexually Transmitted Diseases, 114

Divorce: *Journal of Divorce,* 70

Drugs: *Addictive Behavior,* 11
                    Advances in Alcohol and Substance Abuse, 12
                    Annual Review of Pharmacology and Toxicology, 28
                    British Journal of Addiction, 32
                    Clinical Experimental Pharmacology and Physiology, 40
                    Clinical Pharmacology and Therapeutics, 41
                    Directory of On-Going Research in Smoking and Health, 48
                    Drug Information Journal, 48
                    Hospital Pharmacy, 57
                    Journal of Drug Education, 71
                    Journal of Drug Issues, 71
                    Journal of Studies on Alcohol, 88
                    Medical Letter on Drugs and Therapeutics, 93
                    Smoking and Health, 115
                    Smoking and Health Bibliography, 115

Education: *American Educational Research Journal,* 14
                    Contemporary Education Review, 45
                    Educational Evaluation and Policy Analysis, 49
                    Educational Researcher, 49
                    Educational Technology, 49
                    Education Week, 50
                    Family Life Educator, 52
                    Health Education, 54
                    Health Education Journal, 54
                    Health Education Quarterly, 54
                    International Quarterly of Community Health Education, 62
                    Journal of Continuing Education in Nursing, 70
                    Journal of Educational Research, 71

	Journal of Educational Statistics, 71
	Journal of Nursing Education, 79
	Journal of Nutrition Education, 79
	Journal of Teacher Education, 88
	Media and Methods, 92
	Medical Education, 92
	Nurse Educator, 95
	Patient Education and Counseling, 102
	Phi Delta Kappan, 104
	Review of Educational Research, 114
	Today's Education, 120
Emergency Health:	*Emergency Health Services Quarterly,* 50
	Emergency Medical Abstracts, 50
	Emergency Medicine, 50
	Journal of Emergency Nursing, 72
	Topics in Emergency Medicine, 120
Endocrinology:	*Clinical Endocrinology,* 39
	Clinics in Endocrinology and Metabolism, 43
Enterstomal Therapy:	*Journal of Enterstomal Therapy,* 72
Environmental Health:	*Applied Environmental Microbiology,* 28
	Archives of Environmental Health, 29
	Environment, 51
	Environmental Health Perspectives, 51
	Journal of Environmental Health, 72
	Man and His Environment . . . Journal of Environmental Systems, 91
	Population and Environment: Behavioral and Social Issues, 105
Epidemiology:	*American Journal of Epidemiology,* 17
	International Journal of Epidemiology, 60
Family:	*Child and Family Behavior Therapy,* 37
	Family and Child Mental Health Journal, 51
	Family and Community Health, 52
	Family Life Educator, 52
	Family Planning Perspectives, 52
	Family Practice Research Journal, 52
	Family Relations (Previously *The Family Coordinator*), 53
	Family Therapy, 53
	Family Therapy News, 53
	International Journal of Family Therapy, 61
	Journal of Family Law, 73
	Journal of Family Welfare, 73
	Journal of Marital and Family Therapy, 77
	Journal of Marriage and the Family, 77
	Marriage and Family Review, 91
	Studies in Family Planning, 119
Fitness:	*American Health: Fitness of Body and Mind,* 15
Food:	*Journal of Food Technology,* 73
	Journal of the Science of Food and Agriculture, 86

Gastroenterology: *Clinics in Gastroenterology,* 43
Genetics: *Annual Review of Genetics,* 26
                      Journal of Immunogenetics, 75
Gynecology: *British Journal of Obstetrics and Gynaecology,* 34
                      Clinics in Obstetrics and Gynaecology, 44
                      Journal of Obstetric, Gynecologic and Neonatal Nursing, 80

Hematology: *Blood,* 32
                      British Journal of Haematology, 33
                      Clinics in Haematology, 43
Health Care: *Briefs,* 32
                      Children's Health Care, 38
                      Critical Care Quarterly, 46
                      Dimensions in Health Science, 48
                      Hastings Center Report, 53
                      Health Care Management Review, 54
                      Home Health Care Services Quarterly, 56
                      Law and Medicine and Health Care, 90
                      Merrill-Palmer Quarterly, 93
                      Modern Health Care, 94
                      Social Work and Health Care, 117
                      Topics in Health Care Financing, 121
Health Education: *Health Education,* 54
                      Health Education Journal, 54
                      Health Education Quarterly, 54
                      The Health Educator: A Practical Forum for Health Professionals, 55
                      International Quarterly: Community Health Education, 62
                      Journal of School Health, 85
                      Patient Education and Counseling, 102
Health, general: *Action Newsletter,* 11
                      Imprint, 59
                      Your Life and Health, 59
Health, international: *International Health News,* 59
                      International Journal of Aging and Human Development, 60
                      International Journal of Family Therapy, 61
                      International Journal of Law and Psychiatry, 61
                      International Journal of Mental Health, 61
                      International Journal of Psychiatry in Medicine, 61
                      International Nursing Review, 62
                      International Quarterly: Community Health Education, 62
                      Journal of International Medical Research, 76
                      Journal of Social Psychiatry, 62
                      Social Science and Medicine: An International Journal, 117
Health Law: *American Journal of Law and Medicine,* 17
                      International Journal of Law and Psychiatry, 61
                      Journal of Family Law, 73
                      Journal of Health Politics, Policy and Law, 74
                      Law, Medicine and Health Care, 90

Health Policy: *Health Policy Quarterly,* 55
                        Journal of Health Politics, Policy and Law, 74
Health Services: *International Journal of Health Services,* 60
Health Values: *Health Values,* 55
Homosexuality: *Journal of Homosexuality,* 74
Hospital: *Hospital and Community Psychiatry,* 56
                        Hospital Forum, 57
                        Hospital Pharmacy, 57
                        Hospital Progress, 57
                        Hospitals, 57
                        Hospital Topics, 57
                        Point of View Magazine, 105
Human Ecology: *Human Ecology,* 58
Human Relations: *Human Relations,* 58
Human Services: *Prevention in Human Services,* 106
Hygiene: *Journal of Hygiene,* 75
                        Journal of Tropical Medicine and Hygiene, 89

Immunology: *American Journal of Infection Control,* 17
                        Clinical and Experimental Immunology, 39
                        Clinics in Immunology and Allergy, 43
                        Immunology, 59
                        Infection and Immunity, 59
                        Journal of Allergy and Clinical Immunology, 64
                        Journal of Immunogenetics, 75

Kinetics: *Cell and Tissue Kinetics,* 36

Learning Disabilities: *PsycSCAN: Learning Disabilities and Mental Retardation,* 113
Medicine: *African Journal of Medicine and Medical Science,* 13
                        American Journal of Law and Medicine, 17
                        American Journal of Medical Sciences, 18
                        American Journal of Medicine, 18
                        American Journal of Sports Medicine, 18
                        Annual Review of Medicine, 26
                        British Journal of Medical Psychology, 33
                        British Medical Bulletin, 34
                        Bulletin of the History of Medicine, 34
                        Canadian Medical Association Journal, 35
                        Clinical Nuclear Medicine, 40
                        Clinics in Chest Medicine, 42
                        Clinics in Laboratory Medicine, 44
                        Clinics in Sports Medicine, 45
                        Culture, Medicine and Psychiatry, 46
                        Emergency Medical Abstracts, 50
                        Emergency Medicine, 50
                        International Journal of Psychiatry in Medicine, 61
                        Journal of Behavioral Medicine, 67

	Journal of Holistic Medicine, 74
	Journal of International Medical Research, 76
	Journal of Laboratory and Clinical Medicine, 76
	Journal of Medicine and Philosophy, 77
	Journal of Occupational Medicine, 81
	Journal of the American Medical Association, 65
	Journal of Tropical Medicine and Hygiene, 89
	Laboratory Medicine, 90
	Medical Clinics of North America, 92
	Medical Economics, 92
	Medical Education, 92
	Medical World News, 93
	New England Journal of Medicine, 95
	Oral Surgery, Oral Medicine, Oral Pathology, 100
	Perspectives in Biology and Medicine, 103
	Postgraduate Medical Journal, 106
	Preventive Medicine, 106
	Psychological Medicine, 110
	Psychosomatic Medicine, 111
	Scientific American, 114
	Southern Medical Journal, 118
	Topics in Emergency Medicine, 120
Mental Health:	*Administration in Mental Health,* 12
	Canada's Mental Health, 34
	Family and Child Mental Health Journal, 51
	International Journal of Mental Health, 61
	Occupational Therapy in Mental Health, 99
Mental Retardation:	*American Journal of Mental Deficiency,* 18
	Journal of Mental Deficiency Research, 77
	Mental Retardation, 93
	PsycSCAN: Learning Disabilities and Mental Retardation, 113
Microbiology:	*Annual Review of Microbiology,* 27
	Applied and Environmental Microbiology, 28
Motor Skills:	*Perceptual and Motor Skills,* 103
National Health:	*National Intravenous Therapy Association,* 94
	Nation's Health, 95
Neuro-science:	*Annual Review of Neuro-Science,* 27
	Journal of Neuro-Oncology, 78
	Journal of Neurophysiology, 78
	Spine, 118
Nursing:	*American Journal of Nursing,* 19
	Association of Operating Room Nurses, 30
	Australasian Nurses Journal, 30
	CURATIONIS—The South African Journal of Nursing, 46
	International Nursing Review, 62
	Jamaican Nurse, 63
	Journal of Continuing Education in Nursing, 70

Journal of Emergency Nursing, 72
Journal of Nursing Administration, 79
Journal of Nursing Care, 79
Journal of Nursing Education, 79
Journal of Obstetrics, Gynecologic, and Neonatal Nursing, 80
Journal of Ophthalmic Nursing and Technology, 81
Maternal-Child Nursing Journal, 91
Nurse Educator, 95
Nursing Clinics of North America, 95
Nursing Journal, 96
Nursing Leadership, 96
Nursing Management, 96
Nursing Mirror, 96
Nursing News, 96
Nursing Outlook, 97
Nursing Times, 97
Occupational Health Nursing, 98
Pediatric Nursing, 103

Nutrition: *American Journal of Clinical Nutrition*, 15
Annual Review of Nutrition, 27
British Journal of Nutrition, 34
Dairy Council Digest, 47
Journal of Nutrition, 79
Journal of Nutrition Education, 79
Journal of Nutrition for the Elderly, 80
Nutrition News, 97
Nutrition Reviews, 98
Nutrition Today, 98
Proceedings of the Nutrition Society, 107

Obesity: *Journal of Obesity and Weight Regulation*, 80
Occupational Health: *Journal of Occupational Medicine*, 81
Occupational Health, 98
Occupational Health Nursing, 98
Occupational Therapy in Mental Health, 99
Physical and Occupational Therapy in Geriatrics, 104
Physical and Occupational Therapy in Pediatrics, 104
Ophthalmology: *Investigative Ophthalmology and Visual Science*, 63
Journal of Ophthalmic Nursing and Technology, 81
Journal of Pediatric Ophthalmology and Strabismus, 82
Ophthalmic Surgery, 99
Ophthalmology, 99
Orthopedics: *Clinical Orthopaedics and Related Research*, 41
Orthopedic Clinics of North America, 100
Orthopedics, 100
Orthopedics Today, 101
Otolaryngology: *Clinical Otolaryngology*, 41
Otolaryngologic Clinics of North America, 101

Pathology: *American Journal of Clinical Pathology*, 16
                                    American Journal of Community Psychology, 16
                                    American Journal of Orthopsychiatry, 20
                                    American Journal of Pathology, 20
                                    Oral Surgery, Oral Medicine, Oral Pathology, 100
Patient Care: *Patient Care*, 101
Perinatology: *Clinics in Perinatology*, 44
Physiology: *American Journal of Physiology*, 20
                                    American Journal of Physiology: Cell Physiology, 20
                                    American Journal of Physiology: Endocrinology and Metabolism, 21
                                    American Journal of Physiology: Gastrointestinal and Liver Physiology, 21
                                    American Journal of Physiology: Heart and Circulatory Physiology, 21
                                    American Journal of Physiology: Regulatory, Integrative and Comparative Physiology, 21
                                    American Journal of Physiology: Renal, Fluid, and Electrolyte Physiology, 22
                                    Clinical and Experimental Pharmacology and Physiology, 40
                                    Clinical Physiology, 42
                                    Journal of Applied Physiology: Respiratory, Environmental, and Exercise Physiology, 67
                                    Journal of Neurophysiology, 78
                                    Journal of Physiology, 83
                                    Physiological Reviews, 104
                                    The Physiologist, 105
Primary Care: *Primary Care*, 107
                                    Primary Care: Clinics in Office Practice, 107
Prison Health: *Journal of Prison and Jail Health*, 83
Prostaglandins: *Prostaglandins Bibliography*, 107
Psychiatry: *American Journal of Orthopsychiatry*, 20
                                    American Journal of Psychiatry, 22
                                    Archives of General Psychiatry, 29
                                    Child Psychiatry and Human Development: An International Journal, 38
                                    Culture, Medicine and Psychiatry, 46
                                    Hospital and Community Psychiatry, 56
                                    International Journal of Law and Psychiatry, 61
                                    Journal of Behavior Therapy and Experimental Psychiatry, 68
                                    Journal of Child Psychology and Psychiatry, 68
                                    Journal of Operational Psychiatry, 81
                                    Journal of Psychiatric Research, 84
                                    Perspectives in Psychiatric Care, 103
                                    Psychiatric Clinics of North America, 108
                                    Psychiatric Quarterly: A Publication of the New York School of Psychiatry, 108
                                    Psychiatry: Journal of the Study of Interpersonal Processes, 108
Psychology: *American Psychologist*, 23
                                    Annual Review of Psychology, 28
                                    British Journal of Clinical Psychology, 33

British Journal of Medical Psychology, 33
Contemporary Psychology, 46
Journal of Applied Psychology, 67
Journal of Clinical Psychology, 69
Journal of Community Psychology, 69
Journal of Consulting and Clinical Psychology, 69
Journal of Counseling Psychology, 70
Journal of Personality and Social Psychology, 82
Journal of Psychology, 84
Journal of School Psychology, 86
Journal of Social Psychology, 87
Psychoanalytic Review, 109
Psychological Abstracts, 109
Psychological Bulletin, 109
Psychological Medicine, 110
Psychological Record, 110
Psychological Reports, 110
Psychological Review, 110
Psychology in the Schools, 110
Psychology of Women Quarterly, 111
Psychosocial Rehabilitation Journal, 111
PsycSCAN: Applied Psychology, 112
PsycSCAN: Clinical Psychology, 112
PsycSCAN: Developmental Psychology, 112
Social Psychology Quarterly, 116

Psychosomatics: Journal of Psychosomatic Research, 84
Psychosomatic Medicine, 111
Psychosomatics, 112

American Journal of Psychotherapy, 22
Public Health: American Journal of Public Health, 23
Annual Review of Public Health, 28
Canadian Journal of Public Health, 35
Public Health Reports, 112

Radiology: Investigative Radiology, 63
Radiologic Clinics of North America, 113
Radiologic Technology, 113
Rehabilitation: American Rehabilitation, 24
Journal of Rehabilitation, 84
Religion and Health: Journal of Religion and Health, 84
Research: American Educational Research Journal, 14
American Scientist, 24
Breast Cancer Research and Treatment, 32
Cancer Research, 36
Circulation Research, 83
Clinical Orthopaedics and Related Research, 41
Clinical Reproduction and Fertility, 42
Directory of On-Going Research in Smoking and Health, 48

Educational Researcher, 49
Family Practice Research Journal, 52
Journal of Educational Research, 71
Journal of International Medical Research, 76
Journal of Mental Deficiency Research, 77
Journal of Psychiatric Research, 84
Journal of Psychosomatic Research, 84
Journal of Safety Research, 85
Journal of Sex Research, 86
Milbank Memorial Fund Quarterly/Health and Society, 94
Nursing Research, 97
Phi Delta Kappan, 104
Review of Educational Research, 114
Sex Roles, A Journal of Research, 114
Social Indicators Research, 114
Social Research, 11

Retina: *Retina,* 114

Safety: *Accident Analysis and Prevention,* 11
                       Journal of Safety Research, 85
                       Traffic Safety, 121
Sexuality: *Archives of Sexual Behavior,* 29
                       Birth, 31
                       Journal of Andrology, 66
                       Journal of Homosexuality, 74
                       Journal of Sex Research, 86
                       Journal of Social Work and Human Sexuality, 87
                       Sex Roles: A Journal of Research, 114
                       Sexually Transmitted Diseases, 115
Social Policy: *Journal of Social Policy,* 87
Social Work: *Administration of Social Work,* 12
                       Child and Adolescent Social Work Journal, 36
                       Journal of Gerontological Social Work, 73
                       Journal of Social Work and Human Sexuality, 87
                       Social Casework: The Journal of Contemporary Social Work, 116
                       Social Work in Health Care, 117
Sociology: *American Journal of Sociology,* 23
                       Social Research, 117
                       Sociological Quarterly, 118
Speech-hearing: *American Speech-Hearing Association Journal,* 25
                       Journal of Speech and Hearing Disorders, 87
                       Journal of Speech and Hearing Research, 88
                       Language, Speech, and Hearing Services in Schools, 90
Spine: *Spine,* 118
Surgery: *American Surgeon,* 24
                       Annals of Surgery, 26
                       Clinics of Plastic Surgery, 44
                       Current Surgery, 46

The Journal of Hand Surgery, 74
Journal of Oral and Maxillofacial Surgery, 81
Journal of Thoracic and Cardiovascular Surgery, 89
Ophthalmic Surgery, 99
Plastic and Reconstructive Surgery, 105

Transactional Analysis: *Transactional Analysis Journal,* 121

Urology: *Journal of Urology,* 89
Urologic Clinics of North America, 122

Women: *Women and Health,* 122
World Health: *World Health,* 122